SOS Diet

STOP ONLY SUGAR *Diet*

James A. Surrell, M.D.

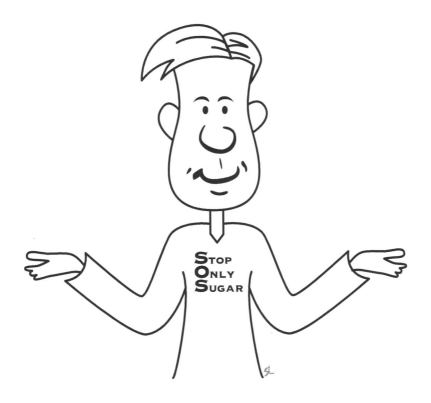

Introducing Sammy SOS
Your SOS Diet Buddy

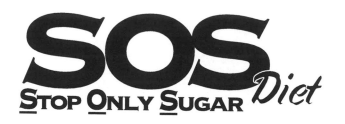

James A. Surrell, M.D.

Layout and Design: Stacey Willey

Cover and Illustrations: Stephanie Lake

Published by

BEAN BOOKS, LLC, Newberry, Michigan

Print Coordination

Globe Printing, Inc., Ishpeming, Michigan

www.globeprinting.net

ISBN # 978-0-9825601-8-1

The information contained in this book represents my personal opinion. It is however, based on 14 years of formal medical education, 20 plus years of clinical practice and experience, and a careful review of many scientific studies. I have no affiliation, formal or otherwise, with any of the companies or products mentioned in this book.

Order on-line at
www.sosdietbook.com

DEDICATION

To my two wonderful children:
Jonathan and Samantha,
for their encouragement, and
especially for just being
who they are.

To our Upper Peninsula family:
Litvok, Mick, Nink, Souse', and Bean

Two of my best friends:
My Father, Dr. Matt Surrell (1910 – 1994)
My Brother, Matt Surrell

You are all so very much appreciated!

Acknowledgements

I owe a very special thanks to my many patients, friends, and colleagues, who continue to enjoy their own success on the SOS Diet, for encouraging me to write this book. They all stressed the importance of my sharing the successful SOS Diet with many others through the medium of this short and simple book. You are all so very special.

Your ongoing support and encouragement is truly appreciated and helped me to persist and complete this work. Your feedback about your personal SOS Diet success stories has been most helpful. Further, your willingness to share your individual success stories clearly speaks to the weight loss success that so many others can now also expect to enjoy.

For their ongoing friendship and encouragement to write this book, I also owe a debt of gratitude to Kevin Vanatta and all my friends at Newberry Motors. I must admit that at this fine automobile dealership, as a colorectal surgeon, I am known as "Tailpipe Doc."

The advice and creativity of the professionals at Globe Printing have been invaluable as we brought the book to print. Their willingness to listen to my ideas, make suggestions, and then help put the short and simple SOS Diet concepts in clear focus has been most refreshing. I remain impressed with their very high quality work.

The truly innovative and creative assistance from Velvet Green Creations web design services has been most impressive. Their talent and expertise is truly appreciated.

A portion of the proceeds from the sale of this book will be donated to various charities.

I sincerely thank you all.

Order on-line at
WWW.SOSDIETBOOK.COM

TABLE OF CONTENTS

FOREWORD (1)

For the better part of my adult life, I have been "pushing maximum density". As you might guess, there were many diets (fad or otherwise) or food/eating plans that I had tried. Some were successful (weight loss) and some were failures (food choices were just nasty). Ultimately, I would lose interest and like so many others, I just could no longer push myself to follow all the way-too-many suggested eating rules. The difficulty for me was that these diet/food plans involved just way too much counting, measuring, weighing, planning, thinking, and generally, they are just way too complicated.

Eventually, in my professional role as a Registered Nurse, I had the good fortune of meeting Dr. Surrell. At the time, I was an all too frequent consumer of regular (non-diet) colas and soft drinks (you know, the ones just loaded with refined sugar). When Dr. Surrell saw what I was drinking, he would gently say, "Do you know how much **SUGAR** is in that bottle?" "But, I **LIKE** sugar", I would respond. Over time, Dr. Surrell would introduce me to the concept of the SOS Diet and convinced me that I could lose weight by merely eliminating refined sugar, so I gave it a try.

The first item to be eliminated was the regular (non-diet) soft drinks which, for only a very short time (about two weeks), was tough for me to do! The minimal short-term suffering was worth it… because, as he said, I began to quickly lose pounds. Next on the "hit list" was pure cane sugar, then white bread, white potatoes and white rice. Well, I lost 83 pounds the first year! The pounds came off and all I was doing was eliminating some everyday food items that, over time, I did not miss at all. No counting, no food logs, no nothing! I didn't ever feel like I was "on a diet". The SOS Diet was the easiest diet to follow and accommodate in everyday life. I could live with that, as I still do today, and so can you.

I continue to enjoy great success on the SOS Diet and I know you will enjoy success as well. Best of luck! - G.M.N.

FOREWORD (2)

Given all of the fad diets, miracle reduced calorie strategies, and weight-loss gimmicks, you might be wondering if Dr. Surrell's SOS Diet actually works, or is it simply another marketing ploy to sell some weight-reduction attention-grabber. Well, I can tell you from dramatic personal experience that it does work. This SOS Diet will offer you both early as well as sustained long-term weight loss.

Doc, as he prefers to be called, and I had been casual acquaintances since the 1980s. But I didn't really get to know him until I began to develop some relatively serious personal health issues including high cholesterol and substantial weight gain. My cholesterol had soared to 270 plus and I had mysteriously accumulated 30 surplus pounds I didn't need nor want! My primary care physician was insistent that I immediately go on a diet, as well as begin taking cholesterol medication.

Shortly thereafter, Doc and I decided to meet for breakfast. He ordered his usual ham and cheese omelet with whole grain toast and peanut butter. I ordered my usual omelet, but with white toast, hash brown potatoes, and I poured on the ketchup and jelly packets. After the server took the order, he tactfully began to describe the health hazards associated with the consumption of the hidden sugar that is so abundant in much of the food the average American consumes daily, including some of what I was having for breakfast. Like so many others, I had no idea of the large quantity of hidden sugar I was ingesting on a daily basis.

As we talked about the hidden sugar in some of my breakfast menu selections, and overall diet, I told him about the disturbing results of my recent visit with the family physician. After listening to my tale of woe, Doc asked if I would be receptive to trying his SOS Diet. Knowing I had to do something, and do it quickly, I responded affirmatively and we met again to implement his simple changes in my diet. As Doc outlined the short and simple SOS Diet for me he emphatically maintained and repeated, "Be patient, and expect to lose about 5 pounds a month. Just stay on the program and you will lose all your excess weight and it will help reduce your cholesterol." He was right... I lost 26 pounds in the first five months, and my cholesterol dropped by 25%.

Prior to the SOS Diet, I had never been successful on any diet. However, with this program, I have been able to make the minor lifestyle change, and I have adhered to the principles set forth in the SOS Diet for the past 10 years. When I began his SOS Diet, I weighed 196 pounds. Now, a decade later, I tip the scales at 162 pounds. Further, my recent blood tests revealed that my cholesterol levels, along with my other medical test results, are all within the normal range. I truly believe that anybody can implement his SOS Diet without having to muddle along with all the complicated food measurements and starve while doing it.

I consider myself very fortunate to be able to enjoy an active lifestyle with relatively minor health issues. Dr. Surrell and the SOS Diet Plan have played a major role in my enjoying ongoing good health. The SOS Diet truly is a short and simple program that will offer you early and sustained weight loss. - R.N.S

Order on-line at
WWW.SOSDIETBOOK.COM

INTRODUCTION

The current national statistics indicate **that the average person in the United States consumes approximately 140 pounds of sugar each year.** Yes, you really did read it right… 140 pounds of refined sugar per person per year! To ingest this much refined sugar annually, we really have to work at it. But we certainly do, as the average American today consumes an astounding 2-3 pounds of sugar each week. **When digested, sugar is stored as body fat.**

This **SOS Diet - _Stop_ _Only_ _Sugar_** book was intentionally written to be a very short book, easy to understand and follow, and is written for the person who wants to be able to follow a very short and simple weight loss program. This practical and proven SOS Diet will allow you to painlessly lose about 5 to 8 pounds per month (60 to 80 pounds per year, or more) and, if needed, will likely allow you to reduce your blood cholesterol levels. The entire SOS Diet is based on the "MISS" Make It Short & Simple concept.

> **By design, these chapters are written
> to be a short and easy read.
> Further, you may read these short chapters
> in any order that you wish.**

It is my strong opinion that other diet programs are way too complicated, with way too many chapters, charts, menus, and they just go on and on and on. These complicated weight loss programs are often like medical text books with multiple chapters and meal planning programs that are nearly impossible to follow with the busy lifestyle that most of us have today. It is very clear to me that this excess detail is the most compelling reason that contributes to the lack of success of most "diets". As you will soon learn, with the SOS Diet, you can forget about counting calories, forget low fat, low cholesterol and low carb diets, forget glycemic index, because it just is not all that complicated!

Nearly every patient, friend, and colleague of mine who start this simple SOS Diet initially came to me with significant frustration about their personal inability to lose any weight. They often state that they had tried nearly every program that they could find on the internet, in bookstores, heard about on the radio, seen on television, or learned about from well-meaning friends and relatives. These many unsuccessful "dieters" have almost always bought into the widely publicized low fat dietary concept. They may have had some initial weight loss success, but they rarely meet their weight loss goal, and quickly become frustrated and overwhelmed with the various programs that are widely available today.

Almost to a person, these unsuccessful "dieters" make this comment. "This or that diet is just too complicated and I cannot get through all of the detailed information to figure out what I can do to lose weight." This frustration then leads to a return to their old lifestyle and even if there was some initial weight loss, they often gain back their initial weight loss, plus extra pounds.

However, with the short and simple SOS Diet, patients not only enjoy **early weight loss success** with the program, but they also have been able to **maintain their desired weight loss over many years.** They almost always tell me that they never, ever felt they were "on a diet". Once again, please know that this book was intentionally written to be short, simple, and easy to understand, so the reader can quickly enjoy the weight loss benefits of the SOS Diet. As you promptly begin to lose your unwanted pounds, you will physically look and feel better, and be on your way to the new and much healthier you.

Before you get started with this short book, let me briefly review (because it is not at all complicated) the only valid and true concepts of what really represents a **rapid and sustained weight loss**.

First, you must understand that any true dietary weight loss involves the loss of body fat. It is essential that you really know what your body does with the refined sugar in your diet. It only knows how to store any excess sugar as body fat! As has been demonstrated by so many of my patients, friends, and colleagues, **rapid**

weight loss comes at the rate of an average of 5 to 8 pounds per month. This obviously will lead to, if needed, a loss of 60 to 80 pounds or more in one year. This loss of 5 to 8 pounds per month is what you should consider to be a rapid weight loss, and it also represents a **true weight loss**. Also, when on any diet, only weigh yourself about every 2 to 3 weeks. Of course, a **sustained weight loss** is one that you can maintain for years. This is the great advantage of the **short and simple SOS Diet** that represents only a **minor dietary lifestyle change** that has been clearly proven to offer both rapid and sustained weight loss.

As a colorectal surgeon, I often prescribe a bowel clean out (prep) for my patients, for a planned colonoscopy examination. The average one day weight loss from a person taking a bowel prep is 8 to 10 pounds! Is this a true weight loss? Of course not! Please be aware of the old saying, "A pint's a pound the world around." Of course, you know that 2 pints makes 1 quart, and 4 quarts make 1 gallon, for a total of 8 pints. Therefore, a gallon of water or similar fluid weighs about 8 pounds, so a gallon of body fluid (mostly water) also weighs about 8 pounds. When a person does a bowel prep, all the stool and liquid normally found in-transit throughout the colon and rectum is removed. Further, there is a significant fluid loss leading to varying degrees of dehydration. This colon cleansing 8 to 10 pound weight loss is a rapid fluid weight loss, but definitely is not a true weight loss at all.

Bottom line... the key to rapid and sustained weight loss can be summed up in just one word – CHOICE. **Choose** the short and simple SOS Diet and you too will soon be enjoying the many healthy benefits of your own successful **rapid and sustained weight loss** program. For multiple examples of "real people", just like you, please keep reading and see Chapter 1, "SOS Diet Success Stories".

With my sincere best wishes for your SOS Diet success,

James A. Surrell, M. D.

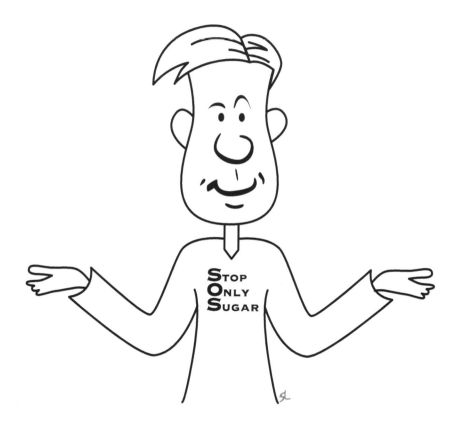

What have you got to lose?

CHAPTER 1

SOS DIET SUCCESS STORIES

REAL PEOPLE (JUST LIKE YOU) SUCCESS STORIES...

The best way to introduce you to the success you can expect from the short and simple SOS Diet is to give you a brief summary of truly representative experiences of various individuals. I have "coded" the initials of these patients, colleagues, and friends to keep them confidential. Read on, believe, and know that you too will soon be enjoying your own personal success on the short and simple SOS Diet.

TYPICAL INDIVIDUAL SOS DIET SUCCESS STORIES

MGW – In late summer of 2008, this 44 year old co-worker and acquaintance came to me with a complaint of a significant weight gain over the past two years. At the time of our initial visit he weighed in at 254 pounds. It was clear that he was very frustrated with his current eating habits and stated he really had developed the habit of snacking on the readily available donuts, cookies and candy. In addition, he drank two or three 20 ounce bottles of non-diet soda pops every day. Like many of us, he grew up with his family eating only white bread. Out of habit, he continued to use white bread for his daily toast and sandwiches. I introduced him to the SOS Diet, and we agreed to spend some time just talking about the SOS Diet with several informal meetings after work. As we reviewed the minor lifestyle change of the SOS Diet, he became more and more enthused about his prospects for success. It seemed to me that he really was motivated and I was impressed at how he really wanted to get off the sugar. His first step was to switch over from the white bread to high fiber, low sugar, whole grain breads for his toast and sandwiches. He later stated it took him about two weeks to get used to only diet soda pop. After this short time, he only drank diet sodas, enjoyed them very much, and now couldn't stand the extra sweet taste of non-diet sodas. He became an avid label reader to avoid all the hidden sugar. Well, at the time of this writing, about 6 months into the SOS Diet, he weighed in at 207 pounds for a total weight loss of 47 pounds. He looks great, feels very healthy, and has repeatedly stated he didn't ever feel like he was "on a diet". Both of us could not be more thrilled with his outstanding SOS Diet results.

MRD – This 49 year old professional colleague had been a calorie counter for many years, and unlike myself and many others, he was very good at keeping track of his caloric intake. He still had a desire for an additional small weight loss, and I of course suggested the SOS Diet. After our brief discussion, I issued the following diet challenge. Just try the SOS Diet for a month, forget the calorie count-ing, and we'll see what happens. He accepted the challenge and we sat down and discussed the basics of the SOS Diet. After we briefly reviewed the "Stop Only Sugar" concept, he stated that it seemed too simple, but he was willing to try it and it would be interesting for him to put it to the test. He agreed to try the SOS Diet for a month, avoid refined sugar, and also follow a high fiber diet, with at least 30 grams of dietary fiber per day. Here are his results. At the end of that one month, he had lost 5 pounds. He also kept close track of his calorie count over that month. Of significant eye-opening interest to him, however, was the fact that **he had not reduced his calorie intake and he still lost 5 pounds in one month.** His calorie intake was the same as it was before the SOS Diet. He did not feel he was "on a diet" at all, but had merely avoided refined sugar and increased his dietary fiber. I just grinned and knew we had another convert to the SOS Diet. I truly appreciated his comment, "We need to forget about counting calories and just Stop Only Sugar!" My return comment to him was, "Welcome aboard."

RNS – This 59 year old male patient came to me with a complaint of having gained 25 extra pounds over the previous several years and his most recent blood cholesterol level was 276, and slowly increasing. He also told me that his primary care physician had been strongly encouraging him to lose some weight, but he had never had much success with "going on a diet". As usual, my first comment was that he was obviously ingesting way too much refined sugar in his diet... and he was not even aware of it. A quick review of his dietary lifestyle revealed that he was indeed consuming large amounts of refined sugar, without even realizing it. Regardless, after our brief visit and discussion to review the SOS Diet, he asked the question I hear nearly every day... "Is that all there is to it?" I gave him my printed information on the SOS Diet. Well, he promised to start the SOS Diet, left me in Michigan's Upper Peninsula to shovel snow, and departed to spend the winter in Florida. I then saw him upon his return about five months later. The following are the actual results that he achieved, and has maintained to this day. Over this initial five month time period, he lost 26 pounds (the typical five pounds per month SOS weight loss result) and felt and looked much better. We then checked his blood cholesterol and it had dropped about 25% in just five short months. Further, he stated that not only did he not miss the sugar... he did not realize that he was ingesting so much hidden refined sugar in his diet. He found the SOS Diet very easy to follow. He has maintained this weight loss over the past ten years by following this simple lifestyle change to avoid refined sugar in his diet. He continues to marvel at how easy it was to not only start the SOS Diet, but how easy it has been to maintain his weight loss.

FCP – This patient came to me several years ago as a 46 year old male who was recently advised he was approximately 90 pounds overweight. He had just been recommended to consider bariatric surgery, as he had failed all other diet programs to lose weight. He had heard about my SOS Diet, and he told me I was his last resort and final hope to lose weight. He had developed significant health issues, including diabetes, joint pain, and elevated cholesterol. He found it difficult to not only exercise, but to even walk short distances. At this time, we discussed the SOS Diet, and I was impressed with his enthusiastic response, as he thought he finally found something he could actually fit into his personal lifestyle. He made the typical comment, "All these diet programs with calorie counting, counting carbs, low fat, and glycemic index checking are just too complicated!" I placed him on the short and simple SOS Diet, and over the course of the next eleven months he lost a total of 80 pounds. He no longer required any medications for his diabetes or for elevated cholesterol. His adult onset diabetes was gone! He began a program of walking as his primary exercise program and stated that he never felt better. Like nearly all other patients, colleagues, and friends who have started the SOS Diet, he just did not realize how much hidden refined sugar he was ingesting in his diet. He also has maintained this significant weight loss and now is enjoying a very healthy lifestyle. He continues to emphasize that he is also enjoying life to a much greater degree than he was previously.

GRL - One of the most interesting patients I have had with the short and simple SOS Diet is a 53 year old female who came to me with the following complaint. She stated that she was now wearing a size 18 dress. Further, for the majority of her adult life, up until approximately five years ago, she had been wearing a size 8 dress. She further lamented the fact that she had tried every popular diet known to human-kind and then verbalized her long list of unsuccessful dietary adventures. Similar to the experience of many others, she did have some very minimal early success with those programs, but found them all to be way too complicated, difficult to understand, and could not follow the many rules. She just could not incorporate the many rules and guidelines into her busy day-to-day lifestyle. As is my usual comment during a conversation along these lines, I advised her that she was merely eating too much refined sugar. She did, in fact, take exception to this and stated that, "I don't eat much extra sugar and I don't believe that is part of the problem." After a review of her day-to-day dietary habits, it became abundantly clear to her that she was indeed ingesting significantly more sugar than she realized. We then briefly discussed the essentials of the SOS Diet. She too asked, "Is that all there is to it?" This initial encounter took place in February. We stayed in touch by phone and she kept me periodically up to date with her progress on the SOS Diet. Then she came back to see me in late December of that same year. I hardly recognized her! She stated that she was now wearing a size 8 dress and that she just had the most delightful Christmas party for her friends and family. The highlight of this Christmas holiday party was all of the desserts and snacks that she prepared using absolutely no sugar. She prepared every sweet snack and dessert with sugar substitutes. Her guests could not rave enough about the delicious treats that she had prepared for them. Since this time, I have seen her on an annual basis and I am pleased to report to you that she is still wearing a size 8 dress. She, too, found the SOS Diet to be not only very easy to get started with, but she also finds it very simple and easy to make this a part of her ongoing lifestyle. She states, "I will never be overweight again, because this program is just too easy to follow. I feel better today than I have in many years. I have the energy that I had when I was in high school." I might add that she obviously felt and looked great in her renewed size 8 wardrobe.

PTN – This female graduate student is a 29 year old individual who came to me with a desire to lose a substantial amount of weight. She stated that her excess body weight was more than 100 pounds and that she, too, had tried numerous diet programs. She found them all to be complicated, too difficult to follow, and she could not consistently fit any of them into her lifestyle. Her frustration was perfectly clear when she stated, "If I hear one more comment about calories, low carb, glycemic index, or low fat, I will scream!" We then had a discussion about the SOS Diet and further discussed at length the amount of sugar in her diet. She, too, was very surprised to learn how much refined sugar was in various products and how certain foods turn into sugar as they are being digested in the body. She admitted that she loved her daily 20 ounce bottle of non-diet cola. Further, she would not drink diet colas because, "Those fake sugars are bad for you." My comment was... "So, you are telling me that the refined sugar is better for you... I don't think so!" I pointed out to her that, in my opinion, there is no credible evidence that sugar substitutes pose any health risks at all! (You will receive the details supporting this in Chapter 7). It was obvious that we had some work to do. I initially pointed out to her that **each 20 ounce bottle of non-diet cola or other non-diet soft drink contains between 15 and 18 teaspoons of sugar.** Imagine this... you sit down, order a large 20 ounce cup of coffee, and then add up to 18 teaspoons of sugar... you wouldn't even dream of doing this, would you? After further discussion, and a review of the SOS Diet, she was excited to follow the simple guide-lines. She now realized how much sugar she was actually ingesting. Similar to the experience of others, she has lost approximately five pounds per month and has found the SOS Diet very easy to follow. She and I are both thrilled with her results of an 87 pound weight loss over 19 months. She also reports that she has a much greater energy level and finds it very easy to continue on the SOS Diet to maintain her significant weight loss. She continues to emphasize to others who comment on her new appearance how easy the program was to initially understand and follow without ever feeling hungry. Because she eliminated refined sugar from her diet, she no longer craved sugar. She was able to completely satisfy her sweet tooth with the ingestion of apples and other low sugar or sugar free products.

MHS – I recently saw this 16 year old high school sophomore. She initially came to me for help with her Irritable Bowel Syndrome (IBS) symptoms of belly cramps, unpredictable bowel pattern, and diarrhea. When we met, she was noticeably overweight. After our initial discussion, it became very apparent that her diet was loaded with refined sugar. The majority of her sugar ingestion was obvious, but some was not. I knew she needed help with her IBS symptoms, but perhaps even more help with her developing childhood obesity. In my practice, I always enjoy seeing patients with IBS, because this condition is very treatable, and refined sugar also worsens the symptoms of IBS. After we discussed her IBS, I gently turned the discussion to her current weight. Knowing that teenagers can be a bit unpredictable, I was delighted to find her quite receptive to a weight loss program. She was fed up with being teased, and was now motivated to lose weight. She said her teachers, parents, and others had talked to her about diet programs, but they were all too complicated and didn't make much sense to her. I assured her that she was not alone in this regard. A brief review of her eating habits quickly revealed that her usual lunch included a 20 or even 32 ounce bottle of non-diet soda pop, and she loved her daily French fries. After this initial meeting she started the SOS diet. Two months later she returned with a 12 pound weight loss. She was thrilled that she finally found a short and simple diet that she could really understand and follow. She also was very pleased that her IBS symptoms were much less frequent and less severe as well. I then explained to her the connection between sugar and various painful abdominal IBS symptoms. Refined sugar is pure carbohydrate made up of carbon, hydrogen, and oxygen. Guess what... two of these become gasses, and it has to go somewhere. Bottom line... sugar adds to the common IBS symptoms of abdominal cramping and bloating. She continues to do well with only minimal IBS symptoms and is continuing her weight loss on the short and simple SOS Diet. This has been very gratifying for both of us.

RNT – This 54 year old man came to see me as a patient after having been on a strict low fat diet for about four months. He had been an acquaintance of mine for years, and if he told me he was strictly following a low fat diet, I knew this to be true. To his surprise and disappointment, he had gained one pound after his four months on his strict low fat diet. He was very healthy, and on no prescription medications. He had experienced about a 20 pound weight gain since his retirement about one year earlier. Of additional concern to this very active gentleman was the fact that he was now experiencing joint pain, which he did not have previously. This new onset of joint pain was significant enough to alter his normally active lifestyle. Further, he advised me that his joint pain had not been present before he started his low fat diet. We initially discussed the simplicity of the SOS Diet. He too was pleasantly surprised at the lack of "rules and regulations" with SOS. We then further discussed that, in my opinion, a strict low fat diet clearly has the potential to cause joint pain and arthritis symptoms. I had observed this in other patients, but it is not too common, perhaps because most people are not very good at following a true low fat diet. I explained that our joints need a certain amount of dietary fat that ultimately will be used to help lubricate our joints. I knew this patient to be a very disciplined individual, and he was anxious to start the SOS Diet. We reviewed the SOS Diet guidelines and I then recorded his current weight. We made a follow-up appointment for him to see me in three months, but advised him to call me anytime with any questions. Upon his return three months later, he had lost 16 pounds. He was enjoying what he called "real food" again, with his favorite breakfast of ham or bacon and eggs, but now with whole grain toast and peanut butter. He also reported that after 3 weeks on SOS, he forgot about his joint pain, as it was completely gone.

TBL – This 53 year old friend of mine came to me after seeing many of our mutual friends and acquaintances enjoy great success on the SOS Diet. I suggested we meet for breakfast the next week-end to discuss the SOS Diet and his current eating patterns. Of course, I wanted to see what he would order for his breakfast and then open the SOS discussion and answer his questions. Yes, I made him pick up the breakfast tab as my professional fee. This gentleman is a very hard working individual and often spends many hours on the road, but is generally back to his home every night. When we met for breakfast, I ordered my usual ham and cheese omelet, whole grain toast with soft margarine, peanut butter and sugar free jam, coffee with Splenda, and water. He also ordered an omelet but loaded his toast with sugar loaded jelly packets and had about 16 ounces of milk. This prompted my discussion about the large amount of sugar in the restaurant jelly packets and the fact that all milk products (including skim, low fat, or whole milk) have about 12 grams of sugar in every 8 ounce serving. We then reviewed his at-home dietary habits, which included drinking lots of milk and high sugar snacks and desserts. I gave him the information on the SOS Diet. He has subsequently decreased, but not totally eliminated, his milk intake and is satisfying his sweet tooth now with apples and the like. He has become a label reader and has lost 20 pounds in just four months. His goal was to lose about 40 pounds in one year and he is well ahead of schedule. Like so many others, he has finally found a short and simple diet program he can follow and never felt like he was ever "on a diet".

KGP – I have known this gentleman for only a short time. He had just heard about the SOS Diet, and this 47 year old man expressed a desire to lose some weight. He was very busy in his job helping to manage the family-owned business and caring for his family. When we met, he was drinking a 20 ounce non-diet cola soft drink. This, of course, prompted me to discuss just how much sugar is hidden in these non-diet soft drinks. We then had a brief discussion of the concept of the short and simple SOS Diet, and it became apparent to me that he was motivated to lose weight. With his busy lifestyle, he did not have time for a complicated diet program. With the SOS Diet, his first step was to switch to only diet soft drinks and he became an avid label reader. Initially, he was surprised to learn just how much sugar is hiding in various fruit juices and many of the so-called "sport drinks". He stopped snacking on high sugar items such as potato and corn chips and, like me, was enjoying dry roasted peanuts, almonds and other low sugar healthy and satisfying snacks. When I saw him recently, he was very pleased to report that he had lost 19 pounds in just the first eight weeks on the SOS Diet. Wow! He remains enthusiastic about his early success on the SOS Diet and found it to be only a very minor lifestyle change, with dramatic weight loss results. He looks great, now has to go buy some smaller waistline pants, and I am almost as excited about his weight loss as he is.

This brief review of the representative experiences of these ten patients and friends are included here to present only a few success stories that are so very typical. Please know that you too will enjoy this kind of success with the SOS Diet. Trust me, as so many others have already done, this will involve **only a very simple and easy lifestyle change** for you.

WALKING – THE SIMPLEST AND BEST EXERCISE FOR MOST OF US

As they lost weight, another benefit experienced by the above individuals and many others, was their increased ability to exercise. Of course, being overweight or obese dramatically limits one's ability and desire to exercise. In my opinion, **one of the best exercises you can do is to just walk**. It is easy on the joints and is also great for your heart, lungs, and muscle tone. Further, it can be a great way to spend some "quality time" with friends and family. Unless you have a physical limitation or medical condition not allowing you to do so, another little trick you can do is to **use the stairs instead of the elevator** for shorter trips between floors. Further, as your personal health status allows, don't always park as close as you can to your destination. It is to your physical exercise advantage to get out of your car and walk a bit further to the mall entrance or store, keeping in mind safety and weather conditions. Try it, you'll like it, and the decreased paint chips and dents on your car doors will just be an added bonus.

Unfortunately, the exercise program for many of us involves roaming around the living or family room of our home looking for the misplaced remote control or our reading glasses. Along these lines, one of my patients once told me that the only way she can get her husband to exercise is to put the television remote control between his toes. Therefore, whenever he wanted to change channels, he would have to do at least one sit-up each time he wanted to get to the remote control! Try it ladies… it might just work… but, being a guy, I would have to say, "Probably not".

It is important to understand that the SOS Diet is based on what I call the "MISS" concept – Make It Short & Simple – and because of this, you will be successful. Once you understand and implement the few short and simple SOS Diet basic concepts, you will be quickly on your way to achieving your desired weight loss. If elevated, you may also reduce your blood cholesterol level. As a result, you will enjoy a lifelong healthier lifestyle and your appearance and self-image will improve. Your predicted lifespan will increase, due to your significantly decreased risk for various overweight and obesity-related illnesses such as diabetes, high blood pressure, heart disease, stroke, breast and colorectal cancers, and others. Further, in only a few months, you likely will have to downsize your wardrobe clothing size... and what fun that will be!

CHAPTER 1
BOTTOM LINE TAKE HOME MESSAGE

The early and sustained long-term effectiveness of the SOS Diet is proven with multiple years of patient experiences. It is very easy to understand, and involves only a **minor lifestyle change**. The short and simple SOS Diet will permit you to easily lose weight as you enjoy many other associated health benefits as you now make very healthy zero or low sugar dietary choices. You will soon increase your ability to exercise and I would encourage you to consider walking as a very healthy exercise activity. **The SOS Diet really works... especially on "Real People" – just like you.**

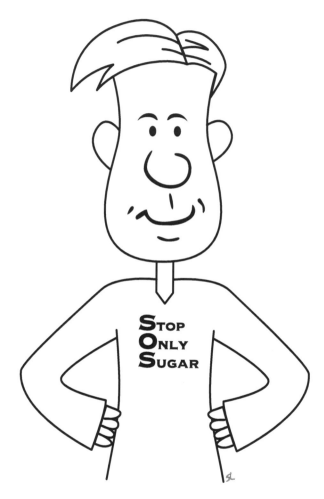

Here's the scientific proof.

CHAPTER 2
SOS DIET MEDICAL RESEARCH

HERE'S THE SCIENTIFIC PROOF

This is a brief summary of the SOS Diet eight week medical research project. These research study results clearly show the effectiveness of the SOS Diet to quickly offer true weight loss and impact on lowering blood cholesterol levels. Now, let's look at the validation of the short and simple SOS Diet with research.

To assess the validity of the SOS Diet, we conducted a two month research project to critically and scientifically assess the effectiveness of the SOS Diet. In addition to assessing their weight loss and cholesterol reduction, we further wanted to gain information from the participants as to how easy or how difficult they found the program to understand and implement with their day-to-day lifestyle. We also wanted to assess the effect of a high fiber diet on feelings of hunger in between meals.

The protocol of this medical research study required that each participant follow the SOS Diet and also follow a high fiber diet with about 30 grams of dietary fiber per day. Further, all study participants were encouraged to drink at least six to eight glasses of water per day, and to especially drink water after consuming dietary fiber.

All volunteer study participants were given written SOS Diet instructions. This was also reviewed in detail by the nurse study coordinator (R.N.) and by me. All their questions were answered to assure their understanding of the short and simple SOS Diet.

A total of seventeen (10 females and 7 males) volunteered to participate in this research project. The only requirement to participate in this 8 week study was to agree to follow the SOS Diet and High Fiber Program, agree to a confidential weigh-in every two weeks, and agree to have their blood serum cholesterol checked before the study, and at the conclusion of the study. All study participant identities remain confidential with regard to identifying the results of any one individual participant. Each participant was given a summary of the study results.

RESEARCH STUDY RESULTS

WEIGHT LOSS RESULTS - Recall that the length of this study was 2 months. **The average weight loss for the 17 participants completing the study was approximately five pounds per month (actually 5.1 pounds).** The range of individual weight loss during this 8 week study period was a high of 16.0 pounds and a low of 2.5 pounds.

CHOLESTEROL LEVEL RESULTS – The laboratory we used for the blood cholesterol levels reports any total cholesterol lab result of <u>201 or greater as elevated</u>, and <u>200 or less as normal</u>. The serum cholesterol levels were elevated in 58% of the participants when they started the study. The post-study cholesterol levels showed that only 31% had elevated cholesterol levels. **In summary, it is very noteworthy that nearly 60% of participants had elevated cholesterol levels at the start of the study, and only about 30% had elevated cholesterol levels at the conclusion of the study.**

FIBER AND FLUIDS - Regarding the addition of fiber and fluids, the study participants reported that they felt no significant hunger for approximately four hours after eating dietary fiber. They also felt satisfied and less hungry for a longer period of time if they ingested approximately twenty ounces of water along with the high fiber meal. This finding is consistent with the fact that dietary fiber is not digested and absorbs fluid while in the digestive system to give one a "full feeling".

RESEARCH STUDY CONCLUSIONS

These study results show that with the SOS Diet, by avoiding or minimizing refined sugar, with increased dietary fiber, participants had an average weight loss of approximately five pounds per month. It is very important to note that, even during this short 8 week study, half of the patients with elevated cholesterol reduced their cholesterol to normal levels. The weight loss and cholesterol reducing effects are entirely consistent with the representative patient experiences and results of the specific individual experiences reviewed in Chapter 1. All study participants stated that the addition of fiber and increased fluids allowed them to go for longer periods of time without feeling hungry at all. They also found the SOS Diet easy to understand and follow, and they planned to continue with the simple lifestyle change of the SOS Diet as their personal ongoing weight management program.

This medical research study confirmed the dramatic and consistent SOS Diet weight loss results. **The study participants lost an average of 5 pounds per month (if needed, will result in a 60 pound weight loss per year)** that has been consistently achieved by so many others who now make the SOS Diet a part of their current lifestyle. Further, as also has been shown by many others on the SOS Diet, **cholesterol levels also dropped**, even during this relatively short 8 week duration of the study.

CHAPTER 2
BOTTOM LINE TAKE HOME MESSAGE

The effectiveness of the SOS Diet is proven with multiple years of patient experiences and in clinical medical research to offer early and sustained weight loss, as well as reduction of blood cholesterol levels. Further, the addition of dietary fiber and fluids allowed participants to eliminate or decrease their feelings of hunger in between meals.

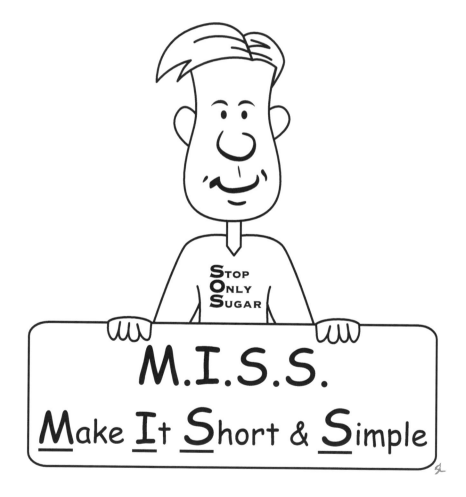

CHAPTER 3
OTHER DIETS ARE WAY TOO COMPLICATED!

INTRODUCING THE "MISS" CONCEPT
MAKE IT SHORT & SIMPLE

About 12 years ago, as I was developing the all-too-common midriff bulge, I decided it was time to lose some weight. Like so many others, I tried all the popular diets. Further, like so many of my patients, friends and colleagues had experienced, **I too was not able to follow the way-too-complicated, low calorie, low carb, low fat, low glycemic index, small portion, too-many-rules, usually unsuccessful popular diet programs**. At this point, I was about to give up and just "get fat" like so many other people. These popular diets didn't work for me and they don't work for most people. As you are painfully aware, they all seem to work well on TV and the internet and the pounds just magically fall off. Isn't it interesting that it just doesn't seem to work that way in real life?

As I reflected on this, I initially believed that in many of today's weight loss programs, something must be missing… but in a moment of profound inspiration, perhaps from above, I realized that just the opposite was true. Most of all this complicated and confusing detail needs to be missing. This was my revelation…

Current popular and often unsuccessful diets today have too many rules and that's the big problem! There is excessive, often confusing and unnecessary information. Bottom line… most of this overwhelming volume of detailed information really needs to be eliminated from these all-too-complex diet programs.

For my patients and friends, nearly all of these complicated diet programs seemed to offer only short-term success, at best. What the public really needs, and we need it now, is a short, easy-to-follow, simple weight loss program that truly represents only a minor life-style change that can be easily maintained over time. Thus, the "MISS" – Make It Short & Simple concept was born... leading to this SOS Diet.

Based on the above enlightenment, I realized that I personally needed a short and simple easy-to-follow diet program. Further, it was apparent from my 14 years of formal medical education and training, along with 20 years of clinical practice in colorectal surgery, digestive health and nutrition, that most diet programs just don't work. I watched so many people unsuccessfully follow the low calorie, low fat, low cholesterol, and low-whatever diet programs that, in my opinion, have way too much complicated information about the role of calories, fat, and cholesterol in your diet.

Further, how many of us have actually purchased a candy bar with a big low fat or reduced fat label glaring at us, perhaps believing it was perhaps a healthy choice... but we really knew it was not! And guess what happened to all that refined sugar in that so-called reduced fat candy bar... that's right, your digestive system dutifully stored it as body fat! What a joke... but the joke's on us! You will soon learn about very tasty and even more satisfying choices for your sweet tooth.

After some homework and research, I became further enlightened and began to realize just how bad refined sugar truly is. For example, did you know that the amount of cholesterol you eat in your diet has only minimal effect on your blood cholesterol levels? It's the sugar that ultimately raises your cholesterol, but much more on this later. However, my big question remained... "How do we get away from all this refined sugar with a short and simple diet program that people will understand, have early and sustained weight loss success, and be able to follow long term, while still satisfying their sweet tooth?" The answer to this question was indeed the beginning of the SOS Diet.

First, I had to prove it to my usual skeptical self. I figured if I could personally have success with a simple program, then I could confidently recommend this program to my patients, friends and others. This was finally decided upon perhaps more out of my personal experience of never being able to lose weight, as well as never being able to control my sweet tooth cravings. After many years of frustration with unsuccessfully counting calories, trying to follow the low carb, low fat, low cholesterol, complicated programs, I just knew there had to be a better way. It was very obvious that we had a growing **obesity epidemic** in this country and elsewhere. **It was also very clear that we all needed a simple and easy way to rapidly start to lose weight and be able to maintain that weight loss over time.**

MY PERSONAL SOS DIET EXPERIENCE

So, here is what I decided to do. For a six week period of time, I would only follow **one simple rule**. **That rule became SOS, meaning Stop Only Sugar**. I would only give up nearly all refined sugar during this six week period of time. My plan was to finally engage in a simple personal program to promote weight loss and health improvement through some **very minor self-discipline**. My first enlightenment was to note that, after only a very short time (about one week), I didn't really miss the sugar and it became readily apparent that this was actually easy to do! I soon figured out that this would mean only a minimal lifestyle change that I knew I could maintain long-term.

At the start of this 6 week exercise, I was about 20 pounds overweight, with a developing "midriff belly bulge", with the usual unattractive "love handles", and a total blood cholesterol level of 221. To this point, my solution was to keep buying larger waist sizes with each new pair of pants... this doesn't sound at all familiar, does it? My suspicion had always been that my sweet tooth was the big culprit, but little did I know how bad refined sugar is for all of us, but much more importantly, how simple it would be to stop all the refined sugar! Wow, was I in for a major personal learning experience! Thus was born the "MISS" concept - Make It Short & Simple.

When I committed myself to start my 6 week program, I finally had become so upset with myself that I really did stick to my plan, and had almost no refined sugar for this period of time. The first enlightenment was that it was so much easier than I thought it would be! I really was a "good boy" and stayed focused on "Stop Only Sugar", while paying absolutely no attention to low calorie, low fat, or low carb concepts.

By following my simple SOS Diet plan, I realized that **I now had to pass all those candy jars on everyone's desk,** full of small wrapped chocolates, jelly beans, mints, and whatever. You all know where they are and what's in those well-meaning but all too commonly found candy jars. Well, about 4 weeks into my new SOS dietary lifestyle, one of my medical office co-workers stopped me and asked me if I was feeling OK, as I looked different and like I was losing weight. She looked at me as though maybe I should get checked over to be sure I did not have some cancer or hidden illness. This moment was so significant to me that I can remember where I was standing in my office at that time. As I thought about her comment, I then also took notice that I was having to tighten my belt one additional notch, and my pants were no longer snug. How could this be? Was it really happening after just 4 short weeks of not eating refined sugar?

When I started this "no sugar" dietary adventure, I made the decision that I would not weigh myself until the 6 week time period was over. This was based on my numerous observations that so many people start their "diet", and then weigh themselves daily, and then just give up after about 3 or 4 days, because they have not "lost weight". This is indeed unfortunate, and I believe it is very unwise to weigh oneself more often than every two to three weeks when one is attempting to lose weight, regardless of the weight loss program. Further, if you drink a lot of fluid before you weigh yourself, you will falsely add to your weight. Always remember how much water actually weighs… "A pint's a pound the world around." Therefore, if my math is correct, a single gallon of water or similar fluid weighs about 8 pounds! As a general guideline to get a true body weight, it is usually best to weigh oneself in the morning, before drinking any fluids.

After being on my SOS Diet for a mere 6 weeks, this is what happened. My first observation was that if I only did not eat refined sugar, my craving for sugar and sweets had significantly decreased. My new "candy bar" now became a daily apple or two, and I snacked "at will" on dry roasted peanuts (which you will learn are very good for you). Well, after only about two weeks, I had a noticeable increase in my overall energy levels, and was sleeping better as well. **When I weighed myself at the end of the six week period, I had lost a total of nine pounds.** Nearly all my family and friends were commenting on my improved appearance, and my clothes noticeably fit and felt better.

Shortly thereafter, I decided to see my internist, and I asked him to draw another blood cholesterol level. He reluctantly agreed, believing it would not be significantly changed from the level noted just two months earlier. **To the surprise of both of us, my cholesterol had dropped from 221 to 183 in just two short months!** This clearly was the result of following my simple SOS Diet (Stop Only Sugar), and never giving one thought to following the low calorie, low carb, low fat, or low cholesterol diet recommendations.

You will hear much more on refined sugar as a significant cause of elevated cholesterol and more details on why much of this low fat diet information is just nonsense! For now, just know that when you eat sugar, your pancreas pours out the enzyme known as insulin. The job of this insulin circulating in your blood is to remove the sugar from your bloodstream, and it stores the sugar as body fat. However, what you really need to know is that this circulating insulin has a very significant secondary side effect… the insulin circulating in your blood tells your liver to manufacture more cholesterol… so, high sugar → high insulin → high cholesterol. Of course, the good news is that the opposite is also true… low sugar → low insulin → low cholesterol… wow, that was easy! You will easily learn much more about the topic of cholesterol in Chapter 5.

Now, what about this "MISS" – Make It Short & Simple concept? It is obvious that for any diet program to offer early and sustained weight loss success, it has to be short, simple, and easy to understand.

Perhaps most importantly, it has to have only a few rules. On many other programs, some of my patients initially enjoyed some weight loss success, but the majority of them fell right back into their previous unhealthy dietary lifestyle, gained all their pounds back, and often more. As I critically reviewed many of the current, very popular and usually expensive weight-loss programs, I became more and more enlightened as to how detailed and complicated they were... no wonder nobody could stick to these weight loss programs!

I remain absolutely convinced, from years of extensive personal, patient, colleague, and friends' experiences, that **the success of any diet program is directly related to the ease with which one can make a simple lifestyle change**. In this regard, I promised myself that this book would have only a minimal number of essential short chapters and would be a "simple and easy read".

As mentioned previously, I studied for 14 years (4 years of pre-med, 4 years of medical school, 5 years of surgery residency, and 1 year of colorectal surgery fellowship) to become board certified in both General Surgery and Colorectal surgery. During these many years, I must admit there was only a small amount of practical nutritional knowledge formally included in our curriculum. In my professional practice I have developed and maintained a keen interest and knowledge base in diet and nutrition. In my practice over the past 20 plus years, I have witnessed first hand the dangers of "nicely overweight", to outright obesity, as it relates to nearly every aspect of one's daily life. Being overweight and obesity results in poor self-image, lack of energy for exercise, personally acquired Type 2 diabetes, elevated cholesterol, increased risk for heart attack and stroke, higher risk for numerous cancers, unnecessary medical and post-operative complications, along with many additional negative health risks from excess body weight.

Well, here I am, after about twelve years of avoiding and not missing refined sugar, weighing about 25 pounds lighter, with low cholesterol, high energy, no prescription medications, and all this after only a very **minor lifestyle change** to easily follow my SOS - Stop Only Sugar diet. The "MISS" Concept – Make It Short & Simple has served me and so many others very, very well.

So, read on, but don't allow too much time out of your busy lifestyle, for what follows will be brief, simple, and straight forward. YOU will be successful with early and long-term weight loss, overall better health, and improved self-image! If I can do it, anybody can do it, and you too will be as successful as I have been. You can do it and will do it... so keep reading.

CHAPTER 3
BOTTOM LINE TAKE HOME MESSAGE

Most diets today are too long and complicated, difficult to understand and even harder to follow. Forget about counting calories, forget low fat, forget low cholesterol, forget glycemic index, and "Stop Only Sugar". The SOS Diet, using the "MISS" concept – Make It Short & Simple – solves all these problems so you too will now be able to enjoy early and sustained weight loss.

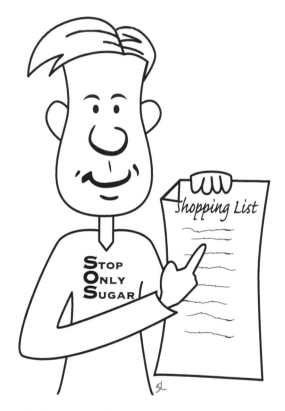

Here's your
SOS Diet
Shopping List

CHAPTER 4
THE SOS DIET ESSENTIALS

NOW HERE'S A NEW CONCEPT FOR BEING ON A DIET - "MISS" – MAKE IT SHORT & SIMPLE

It is important for you to know that I developed the SOS Diet with a well studied and focused understanding of the many, significant health problems that may occur as a result of the ingestion of refined sugar. The bad news is that childhood and adult obesity in the United States and elsewhere now represents perhaps our most significant challenge to health care. Further, know that the ingestion of refined sugar is the overwhelming cause of the problem of childhood and adult excess weight and obesity, with the resulting childhood and adult diabetes, elevated cholesterol, heart disease, stroke, increased risk of breast, colon, and other cancers, increased infection rates, dental cavities, lack of energy, and on and on and on. The current Centers for Disease Control and Prevention (CDC) statistics show that 66% of adults aged 20 and older in the USA are considered overweight or obese. Further, the number of overweight and obese children and adolescents aged 2 through 19 years also remains very high at 32%. In other words, about 2/3 of adults and 1/3 of children in the USA are overweight or obese! Unfortunately, the majority of overweight and obese children continue this health problem into adulthood.

So, where's the good news? The **good news** is that this significant overweight and cholesterol problem affecting so many of us has a proven solution... the SOS Diet. The reason for this good news is that you now have a short and simple diet, involving only a minor lifestyle change. This is a diet for all of us who just can't follow a diet, as has been clearly demonstrated by the success stories noted in

Chapter 1. Further, the SOS Diet offers you both early and sustained weight loss over many years.

All of my many patients, friends, and others who successfully follow the SOS Diet marvel at the simplicity and ease of understanding the SOS Diet minor lifestyle change. Next, they marvel at how easily and quickly they start to drop pounds, lose their craving for refined sugar, have more energy, sleep better, and finally are able to lose their unwanted pounds. More importantly, they MAINTAIN their desired weight loss! They all tell me how they are very impressed with the "MISS" concept – Make It Short & Simple. Almost to a person, they comment, "I don't feel like I am on a diet… it's just too easy."

Let me again emphasize how important it is for you to always keep in mind what SOS really stands for… "Stop Only Sugar". Based on the rapid and sustained weight loss of so many people, further confirmed by our medical research, it is clear that the SOS Diet is so successful because of the "MISS" concept (Make It Short & Simple). They enjoy success by shedding unwanted pounds, and this is followed by a **delightfully positive impact on their self-image**. This improved self-image is based not merely on their improved appearance, but more importantly, on their significant personal success not only to choose to start the program, but to choose to continue the easy-to-follow SOS Diet. They have more energy, their doctors may have them taking fewer medications, and their previous significant risk for obesity, diabetes, heart disease, stroke, vascular disease, various cancers, infections, and other serious illnesses is greatly decreased.

SOS DIET SUCCESS REQUIRES THAT YOU READ LABELS!

First and foremost, **you must avoid or minimize refined sugar**. This cannot be emphasized too much, and is the **key to your success**. Further, know that the ingestion of refined sugar is the primary cause of a person's excess weight and may have a significant impact leading to elevated cholesterol. I cannot emphasize enough how you **must**

become a food label reader. However, now you **read the label to learn the sugar content, and also check for the dietary fiber** (more on this simple fiber concept later).

With regard to food labels, you must remain aware of the following. Some food and drinks do not list sugar content, and may list only carbohydrates. If you do not see the sugar content on the label, then check for carbohydrates and consider this to be sugar content.

The first example of where the carbohydrates should be considered as sugar is the **labeling on potato chips and corn chips**. The labels on these popular types of snacks will show zero grams of sugar. However, since these snacks are rapidly converted to sugar when they arrive in your stomach, they are digested as sugar, then stored as body fat. You should consider potato chips and corn chips as high sugar... relax, and know there are many other zero sugar or low sugar healthy snacks (such as dry roasted peanuts) that you will enjoy on the SOS Diet.

Another example of this would be the **labeling on beer** that shows no sugar, but does show the grams of carbohydrate... these grams of carbohydrate should be considered as refined sugar! Don't panic... as you will see below, the so-called "light beers" generally have a low sugar content and are OK (in moderation) on the SOS Diet. **A reasonable guideline is to consider a "light" beer has about 4 times less sugar than a regular "non-light" beer.** A few examples of the very low sugar brands of "light beer" are noted below in your SOS Diet "Shopping List".

Review the following two short and simple lists. Table 1 is the SOS Diet "No-No" List and Table 2 is your SOS Diet "Shopping" List. You must AVOID or minimize all of the items following on the "No-No" List, as they are loaded with refined sugar, or are converted to sugar in the process of digestion (such as potatoes and corn). Further, as you soon will become aware, you will really enjoy all the great tasty healthy foods on the "Shopping" List. **Take note that the SOS Diet "Shopping" List is much longer than the "No-No" List!**

TABLE 1 - SOS DIET "NO-NO" LIST
(HIGH SUGAR CONTENT)

○ **All sugar candy** (just relax and keep reading as it will be much easier than you think…)

○ **All desserts made with refined sugar** (again, don't panic, more suggestions later…)

○ **White bread** (whole grain or whole wheat breads are OK, but whole grain is better)

○ **White flour pastry,** donuts, and rolls (high fiber, low sugar bran muffins are OK)

○ **White potatoes and potato chips** because they are starch, and starch is converted to sugar so this is like eating sugar… (So, the potato chips and French fries are only for "once in a while"…)

○ **White rice**

MEMORY AID – "If it's white, it's just not right!" – So generally avoid white bread, white pastry, white potatoes, and white rice… they just turn to sugar in your body.

○ **Corn and corn chips…** (Occasional popcorn is OK, but not to excess… limit yourself to 2 or 3 times a week, or when at the movies… remember, corn gets stored as sugar when digested)

○ **Beets** (lots of sugar here…)

○ **Fruits - Grapes** are very high in sugar, so use sparingly. Nearly all **canned fruits** are loaded with sugar…, check the label!

○ **Dried Fruits - a cup of raisins has 116 grams of sugar** so always check the label on any dried fruits, due to high sugar content

○ **Honey** is pure sugar (you won't miss it… you really are not a honey bee, are you…?)

○ **Pancake and waffle syrup** and other high sugar condiments such as molasses, barbecue sauces, and the like

○ **Carrot Sticks as a snack item** are to be avoided due to the high sugar content

⊘ **Salad Dressings** – often those labeled as low fat have lots of sugar… so be sure to read the label for sugar content on these and other condiments

⊘ **Ketchup** - one tablespoon of ketchup has 4 grams of sugar

⊘ **Jams and Jellies** are loaded with sugar … usually about 12 grams per tablespoon, or in a small restaurant packet

⊘ **Fruit Juices** - lots of sugar in most - here are the grams of sugar per one cup (8 ounce) serving of various juices – grape = 40, apple = 27, orange = 21, grapefruit = 18, tomato = 9, and V-8 Brand = 8, (so read the juice label and choose wisely!)

⊘ **Milk** (white) contains about 12 grams of sugar per 8 ounce cup, regardless of whether it is whole, reduced fat or skim milk, **so just do not use to excess** and note that chocolate milk has about twice as much sugar as white milk with 24 grams of sugar per 8 ounce cup. Know also that soy milk has about half the sugar of cow's milk at about 6 grams of sugar per 8 ounces

⊘ **Yogurt with high sugar content**… you really need to be a label reading detective here, because all yogurts are not created equal. For example, a small six ounce serving of yogurt may have up to 33 grams of sugar! Most of the so-called low fat varieties almost always have about 27 grams of sugar, so be wary, and wisely choose the lowest sugar yogurt

⊘ **All non-diet soft drinks**… and recall that many so-called "sport drinks" are high in sugar content. Note that **all diet soft drinks and most electrolyte-enhanced water drinks are OK**, but always check the label on these drinks for sugar content

⊘ **Sweet wines** (dry wines are OK, but check the label for sugar content and always use good sense with regard to any alcohol use…)

⊘ **Regular "non-light" beer** usually has a high sugar content and count the carbohydrates in beer as sugar… you may be surprised at the amount of sugar in these "non-light" beers, and recall that regular "non-light" beer has about 4 times as much sugar as in the "light" beers

TABLE 2 - SOS DIET "SHOPPING" LIST

(ZERO TO LOW SUGAR CONTENT)

BREADS, CEREALS, CRACKERS, AND GRAIN PRODUCTS

☑ **Whole grain and whole wheat** breads and pastry are very good for you, but read the label and **always choose the lowest sugar and highest fiber breads**. There are many low sugar, high fiber breads available. For example, two slices of Brownberry brand Multigrain "Carb Counting" brand bread has 6 grams of fiber, zero grams of sugar, and 10 grams of protein. Two slices of Sara Lee brand "45 Calorie" wheat bread has only 2 grams of sugar, along with 5 grams of fiber and 6 grams of protein… either will be a very healthy SOS Diet choice

☑ Here are two of my personal favorite grain products: 1) **Thomas' brand "Light" muffins** (less than 1 gram of sugar and 8 grams of fiber per muffin) and 2) Thomas' plain "100 Calorie" bagels (less than 1 gram of sugar and 4 grams of fiber per bagel)

☑ **Original Fiber One** brand cereal has **14 grams of dietary fiber and zero sugar** in a half cup serving, and if you don't want to have it as a cereal with milk, use it as your croutons on your salad (but only with low-sugar salad dressing, of course**). Use the milk sparingly on your cereal**, and if it suits your taste buds, know that soy milk has about half the sugar of cow's milk with about 6 grams of sugar per 8 ounces, instead of 12 grams per 8 ounces

☑ Wheat Thins brand "Fiber Selects" 5-Grain crackers with only 4 grams of sugar and 5 grams of fiber in a generous serving of 13 crackers, and other taste varieties available

☑ Triscuit brand crackers with zero grams of sugar and 3 grams of fiber in a serving of 6 crackers

MEAT, FISH AND CHEESES

☑ Nearly any amount of beef, ham, pork, bacon, chicken, turkey, and fish

☑ Most varieties of salami, bratwurst, hot dogs, lunch meats, most cheeses (but if you make a sandwich only use the breads as noted above)

☑ Nearly all cheeses are fine, and serve as an excellent source of calcium and high quality protein that will satisfy your appetite... my personal favorites are Colby, Swiss, and Cheddar that I often enjoy with some slices of turkey or ham, or in a meat and cheese sandwich

☑ Win Schuler's brand original cheddar cheese spread with only 2 grams of sugar in a 2 tablespoon serving... many other cheese spread brands are available and are very tasty with low sugar and high protein, but, as always... check the label for sugar content

DAIRY PRODUCTS

☑ All the eggs (with or without ham or bacon) you want, and omelets, but stay away from the side order of potatoes or white bread toast. You must NOT use the high-sugar little jam and jelly packets in restaurants, so just ask for peanut butter and also ask for the sugar free little jam or jelly packets instead

☑ Recall that soy milk has about half the sugar of any variety of cow's milk, but use whatever suits your taste buds, but not to excess

☑ Most cheese varieties are very low or zero sugar, zero trans fats, high protein, high calcium, but this varies, so always check the label

SNACKS AND DESSERTS

☑ Peanuts, almonds, cashews and various nuts are great

☑ Planters brand dry roasted peanuts - one generous serving of about 40 peanuts has only 2 grams of sugar, 2 grams of fiber and 7 grams of protein... this is my favorite snack item...

☑ Emerald brand Cocoa Roast Almonds have only 1 gram of sugar, but with 3 grams of dietary fiber in a one ounce serving of this great tasting mildly sweet snack

☑ Sunkist brand Gourmet Oven Roasted Almonds with Sea Salt also have only 1 gram of sugar and 3 grams of dietary fiber in a one ounce serving, with a great mildly salty taste

☑ Any sugar free candy (readily available in most stores or on-line today)

☑ Sugar free desserts... (readily available for purchase, or just make them with Splenda... and the only change you will notice will be in your shrinking waistline...)

CONDIMENTS AND SPREADS

☑ Peanut butter (smooth or crunchy) - Jif, Skippy or Peter Pan brands are very tasty with low sugar... as a large 2 tablespoon serving has only 3 grams of sugar, 2 grams of fiber, zero trans fats, and 7 grams of protein... **peanut butter is my favorite "health food"**

☑ **Any sugar free jams and jellies**... Smucker's brand is my personal favorite, and don't forget to ask for the little sugar free jam or jelly packets in the restaurant

☑ Any soft margarine... some brands of butter and hard margarine may still have trans fats so just check the label

☑ Use only sugar free pancake and waffle syrup and low sugar condiments... read the label

☑ Salad dressings should be low sugar or sugar free such as vinegarette or oil and vinegar – "Newman's Own" brand varieties are great... but be sure to read the label for the sugar content and just ignore the low fat or reduced fat labeling often found on these items

☑ Look for the sugar free varieties of items such as ketchup or cocktail sauces

FRUITS, VEGETABLES AND JUICES

☑ **Apples** are a great "sweet tooth" snack, and are my favorites... just forget the natural sugar in the apples and recall that the dietary fiber is a nutritional bonus...

☑ **Oranges and Bananas** are OK, but no more than one a day or less

☑ **Green vegetables and beans** are great, but watch out for the added sugar in many baked bean preparations, or make your own with Splenda

☑ Carrots are nutritious, so use on salads, and only as an **occasional** snack, but not to excess, due to high sugar content

☑ V-8 juice or tomato juice are the juices lowest in sugar, as they both have about 1 gram of sugar per ounce... just don't fall for the "no added sugar" labeling on some juices, as they may be very high in sugar... so read the label for the sugar content on all juices before you choose to buy

BEVERAGES, INCLUDING ALCOHOLIC VARIETIES

☑ Use only sugar substitutes for your coffee or tea and it's OK to add some milk, half & half, or cream

☑ **All diet soft drinks** and most electrolyte-enhanced water drinks are OK, but be careful to check for sugar in some of the so-called "sport drinks" (hey, how many times do I have to say it... check the label for sugar content)

☑ "Dry" wines or "light" beers - the light beers are OK, due to much lower sugar content, and recall that regular "non-light" beers have about 4 times the sugar of the so-called "light" beers. Miller Lite, Miller MGD 64, Busch Light, and Michelob Ultra are examples of brands with low sugar content, but always read the label and remember you have to count the beer carbohydrates as sugar. (I have to tell you this one that made me almost fall off my chair. One of my patients said she could not give up her nightly glass of sweet wine, so she purchased dry wine and simply added a packet of Splenda to each glass – please don't you dare tell them at the winery... they may not approve!)

Of course, you will find many other zero or very low sugar items that will completely satisfy your personal taste preferences. Like so many others, as you bring this simple dietary lifestyle change into your day-to-day dietary pattern, you will enjoy early and sustained true weight loss, all without ever feeling like you are "on a diet".

Hey Doc, what about calcium? Good question, my SOS friend, and I'm glad you asked. As you know, milk is nutritious and an excellent source of calcium. However, milk (including skim and the low fat varieties) does contain 12 grams of sugar per 8 ounces, so use good SOS Diet judgment with regard to the amount of milk you consume. I use a small amount of milk on my Original Fiber One cereal, but not to excess. It is generally recommended that adults have about 1200 mg. of calcium every day. I certainly believe in taking calcium supplement tablets, and I take two of the 600 mg. calcium with vitamin D tablets every day. Further, cheese can be an excellent source of calcium.

Please review and follow these suggestions regarding the necessity of washing any **organic foods** very, very carefully. Basically, organic food products are generally defined as foods grown without any pesticides, but are still usually fertilized with manure. Organic foods may come from other countries, and the source of the manure may not be known. I don't happen to eat organic foods, but I have no personal preference or recommendation for any person to use or not to use organic foods. That is your choice. However, if you choose to do so, be certain to carefully wash your organic foods, especially vegetables. They must be washed very thoroughly, as they may well have various types of viable "natural" organisms that must not be ingested.

Let me wrap up your "SOS Diet Essentials" with an example of the dramatic impact various **dietary choices** can have on your sugar intake, with high sugar leading to added pounds and elevated cholesterol.

GREAT SOS DIET CHOICE

1) Your own creation of SOS Diet "Trail Mix" with 3 cups Planters brand Dry Roasted Peanuts and 1 cup Original Fiber One brand cereal… a generous serving of about 120 dry roasted peanuts mixed with the Fiber One Cereal is very filling and satisfying.

2) A 20 ounce <u>diet</u> soft drink, or large coffee, or with 2 or 3 packets of Splenda brand sugar substitute and/or creamer has zero sugar.

Total sugar = **6 grams of sugar** in this great filling snack!

Next, imagine you look across the room and see a friend of yours who decided to have the following snack instead - and this should be a real eye opener...

VERY POOR SOS DIET CHOICE

1) A medium size (four ounce) bag of caramel corn has a whopping 160 grams of sugar!

2) A regular (non-diet) 20 ounce soft drink has about 80 grams of sugar.

Total sugar = **240 grams of sugar** in one little snack!

Remember, in life and on the SOS Diet, it's all in the choices we make. Follow the SOS Diet choices and you are now on your way to early and sustained weight loss, lower cholesterol, and better health!

The SOS Diet involves the essential concept of eliminating or significantly decreasing the amount of refined sugar in your diet. It is designed to be short and simple, easy to understand, and involves only a minor lifestyle change. As you become a devoted label reader, you will easily be able to avoid or significantly decrease the amount of refined sugar in your diet. This will, of course, lead to the renewed slimmer and healthier you.

CHAPTER 4
BOTTOM LINE TAKE HOME MESSAGE

To lose weight, limit your refined sugar intake to no more than 20 grams per day. Of course, less than 20 grams per day will result in more rapid weight loss. To maintain your current weight, limit your refined sugar intake to no more than 30 grams per day. Further, as so many others have found, after a very short time you won't miss the refined sugar at all.

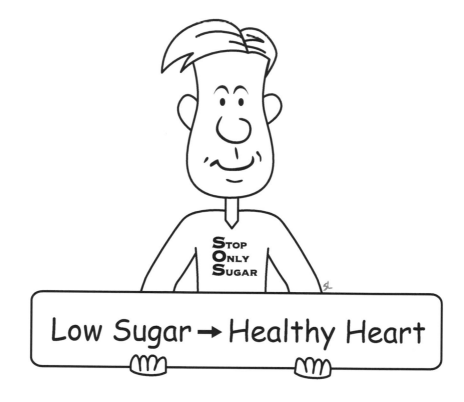

CHAPTER 5
CHOLESTEROL AND THE
LOW FAT DIET MYTH

In the late 1890's in the United States, the average consumption of sugar was only about 4 to 5 pounds of sugar per person per year. As a result of the very low sugar diet, obesity was uncommon. Cholesterol was not yet a "dirty word" and it obviously had not yet been discovered as a necessary biochemical substance in our human metabolism.

Compare the 1890's sugar consumption to our current statistics indicating that **the average person in the United States consumes approximately 140 pounds of sugar each year. The average American consumes an astounding 2-3 pounds of sugar each week.** This is easily understood when we look at so many of our food choices today loaded with highly refined sugars in the forms of sucrose (table sugar), dextrose (corn sugar), and high-fructose corn syrup. Frankly, sugar is hiding everywhere in our popular foods. When they start the SOS Diet, most people are shocked to learn how much refined and hidden sugar they actually take into their bodies every day.

Why all the fuss about refined sugar, you ask? Just look at the dramatic and major negative health impact of this high refined sugar diet. It has been variously estimated that a high sugar diet may account for as many as 150,000 annual heart disease deaths in the USA. In addition to significant heart disease, high sugar intake leads to child and adult obesity, child and adult diabetes, dental cavities, overall increased risk of cancer, increased risk for various infections, risk for stroke, mood swings, poor self image, and on and on and on. In other words, we are literally killing ourselves with our very unhealthy and widespread high refined sugar diet.

There are multiple studies from Europe and elsewhere that have reviewed the long-term results of low fat diets, for periods of time up to a decade. As has been my clinical experience, they report that the impact of a low fat diet on lowering blood cholesterol levels is very minimal, if at all. These results are consistent with the fact that the vast majority of the cholesterol in your body is manufactured in your body, and does not come from dietary fat and cholesterol. Let's face it, these low fat, low cholesterol diets are, for the most part, not effective in reducing your cholesterol. We now know that trans fats are bad and unsaturated fats are good. But there are conflicting reports on whether saturated fats are good or bad. However, do not fall for all this low fat or reduced fat labeling, because these products are often loaded with refined sugar... and that may well send your weight and your cholesterol through the roof. **Again, always check the label for lowest sugar and highest fiber, because these are two of the healthiest dietary choices you can make.**

Now, why am I making such a big deal about refined sugar and cholesterol? Why is there no emphasis on a low fat diet? What about limiting the amount of ingested cholesterol in my diet? Why are so many people following a strict low fat diet, not losing any weight, some having joint pains, not lowering their cholesterol and still needing their cholesterol-lowering prescription medications? Of course, there are people who need these effective cholesterol-lowering medications, and that decision must remain with you and your physician. Further, these medications are also not without side effects. **However, you should never, ever start or stop prescription medications without consulting with your physician or health care provider! This is so important, so let me emphasize it one more time... never, ever stop any prescription medication without first consulting with your physician or other health care provider.**

Without question, there are individuals who have **elevated cholesterol due to hereditary factors**, and these people are often identified by their health care providers based on a significant family history of heart disease. Fortunately, however, these hereditary causes of elevated cholesterol are uncommon. For example, the condition known as Familial Cholesterolemia (FC) occurs in only 1 in 500 people, or only 0.2% of the population. There is ongoing research and debate regarding hereditary factors and elevated cholesterol, as well there should be. Individuals with hereditary factors affecting their blood cholesterol may or may not be obese or overweight at all, may not ingest significant amounts of refined sugar, and they still have elevated cholesterol. Of course, these individuals should never personally use tobacco, and should never allow themselves to be exposed to the dangers of second-hand smoke, as noted in Chapter 12. These individuals may well need, and likely will benefit from, prescription cholesterol-reducing medications, as recommended by their health care providers. Further, they may also benefit from the SOS Diet, to further help lower their cholesterol and triglyceride levels. **Whenever there is a significant family history of heart disease, in the absence of obesity and/or tobacco abuse, it is strongly recommended that this be discussed at length with your personal health care provider. This is yet another example of the importance of knowing your family medical history.**

So, let's get on with a brief discussion of these various topics and give you a **short and simple explanation of the relationship between refined sugar, high fiber diets, and blood cholesterol levels.**

No one would dispute the well-established medical fact that cardiovascular disease is often related to elevated blood cholesterol levels. We are still learning about the HDL (good cholesterol) and LDL (bad cholesterol) and other subtypes, and research is ongoing. However, for our discussion here, let's accept the fact that if your personal blood cholesterol is less than 200, your total cholesterol to HDL ratio is 4.0 or less, and you do not have a significant personal or family medical history of heart disease, you generally would not be considered to be at high risk for cholesterol-related heart disease.

Now let's review the **cholesterol eye-opener** for most people. Finally, it is now being appreciated is that these increased rates of cardiovascular disease are linked to increased sugar intake. This sugar and heart disease association was reviewed in *Circulation - Journal of the American Heart Association* in August of 2009. **Further, many respected studies now show that dietary fat and dietary cholesterol intake are now believed to be minimal factors in raising your blood cholesterol levels.** Table sugar (sucrose) causes an increase in triglycerides, increased total blood cholesterol, increased LDL (bad) cholesterol, and decreased HDL (good) cholesterol, or the worst case for each of these four factors. What follows is a short and simple discussion of how refined sugar may well be the dietary culprit most related to your elevated blood cholesterol level.

This is so important that you understand this concept. So, let me say this one more time, with emphasis…

Very important… the amount of dietary fat and dietary cholesterol that you eat are only minimal factors in raising your blood cholesterol levels. Know this… your elevated cholesterol is more related to eating refined sugar!

So, what happens when you eat refined sugar? The human body can do only one of two things with ingested refined sugar… it will either use it as instant energy (very unlikely, unless you go out and run around the block 7 times after you eat a candy bar), or it will store it as body fat (about 99% likely). When you eat refined sugar, this promptly causes the pancreas to start working overtime to pour out insulin, resulting in a dramatic increase in the insulin levels in your bloodstream. The circulating insulin grabs the sugar and stores it as body fat.

A not-so-well publicized **side effect of circulating insulin** is that it causes the liver to actually manufacture more cholesterol. So, here's the sugar/cholesterol connection: you eat excess sugar → the pancreas releases more circulating insulin → insulin stores the sugar as body fat → the circulating insulin causes the liver to manufacture more cholesterol → blood cholesterol level goes up above safe and normal levels → risk of heart disease goes up, and this is all because of the sugar you eat! **To summarize, in the same manner that the**

pancreas (your internal insulin factory) pours out the insulin in response to the sugar you eat, the liver (your internal cholesterol factory) pours out cholesterol in response to the circulating insulin. Health care professionals that care for diabetics have noted for years that when an individual is started on insulin, they must monitor the patient's cholesterol levels, which may well go up significantly.

A SHORT COURSE IN CHOLESTEROL BIOCHEMISTRY

This will be very brief, short and simple, because when I took biochemistry in medical school, they also gave me credit for studying a foreign language. Of course, it can get complicated, but it certainly won't be here. Please keep reading.

In the cells of the human body, production of cholesterol is tied to the function of an enzyme called 3-hydroxy-3-methyl-glutaryl-Coenzyme-A Reductase (HMG-Coenzyme A Reductase), and thank goodness this is abbreviated as the enzyme HMGR. Come on, Doc, why would I care about this boring biochemistry HMGR enzyme stuff? Well, all you need to know is that certain chemical substances block HMGR, and decrease the production of cholesterol. Other chemical substances promote HMGR, and increase the production of cholesterol. Keep reading.

About two decades ago, the very smart pharmaceutical company biochemists developed a medication to block HMGR, to result in lower blood cholesterol. As a group, these medications are called "statins", and they are now among the largest selling prescription medications world-wide. Just a few examples of brand names of "statins" include: Lipitor, Mevacor, Crestor, Zocor, and many others. By blocking HMGR, these "statins" are very effective in lowering cholesterol, but, like most medications, they do have side effects.

O.K. Doc, what chemical substance promotes HMGR? The answer is. . . insulin. In the human body, the pancreas produces insulin in response to eating sugar. With increased refined sugar in your diet, this quickly leads to increased levels of insulin. This natural human hormone insulin promotes HMGR and therefore has the undesired effect of raising your blood cholesterol. Too much sugar → too much insulin → insulin promotes HMGR → too much cholesterol.

Now you know why the most significant dietary impact on elevated blood cholesterol is too much sugar in the diet, leading to elevated insulin levels that result in excess cholesterol production. This is why so many of my friends, patients and colleagues on the SOS Diet not only quickly lose the pounds, but they also lower their blood cholesterol.

WHERE DOES YOUR CHOLESTEROL COME FROM?

Various authorities will not completely agree on the exact percentages, but about 75% to 85% of the cholesterol in your body is actually manufactured in your body, primarily in the liver. Based on my clinical experience and the lack of results of a low cholesterol diet, I believe that only about 15% of our cholesterol comes from dietary fat and dietary cholesterol. Perhaps by now you are sitting on the edge of your seat wondering if cholesterol truly is this mean and evil substance you have been told it is. No, it is not. If cholesterol was so "bad" for us, why would our liver manufacture cholesterol? **Well, cholesterol is an essential building block component of our necessary human hormones, human steroids, vitamin D, bile, and is found in the walls of every one of the 50 trillion or so cells in the human body. Know this... we cannot live without cholesterol... it is not the bad guy it has been made out to be. So, if we do not ingest enough cholesterol, our body manufactures it for us.** This little gem of information is not well publicized, so please appreciate that cholesterol is a naturally occurring and necessary human biochemical substance. As one of my medical school professors (way ahead of his time) so aptly put it, anything that is used by the body to manufacture our human sex hormones can't be all bad!

So, here's the SOS Diet low sugar → low cholesterol connection. You limit your dietary intake of refined sugar and therefore, you release much less insulin from the pancreas, the liver is not manufacturing excess cholesterol, and, as happened to me and so many others, you likely will drop your cholesterol while you drop your excess pounds. The decline in cholesterol is almost a free bonus as you shed your unwanted pounds by following the SOS Diet. The SOS Diet eliminates all the complicated and unnecessary dietary information that you don't need... and gives you all the simple and effective nutritional information you really do need. This is presented to you in keeping with the "MISS" concept, Make It Short & Simple.

As we all are so painfully aware, over the past 2 to 3 decades, you cannot watch T.V., listen to the radio, go on-line, or read a magazine or the newspaper without being bombarded with information about the evils of fats in your diet. Thus was born the concept of the low fat diet. So I ask, if all these widely publicized low fat diets were at all effective, why is obesity and diabetes such a true health care epidemic in our society?

I am certain you have noticed the extensive and growing low fat, reduced fat, light, and other labeling on so many of our foods. Don't be fooled... read the label for sugar content! In my significant experience, these low fat diets are ineffective and just don't work.

When looking at fats in your diet, you need to know that the unsaturated fats are considered to be the "good fats" as they have the effect of lowering total cholesterol and LDL cholesterol, and raising the HDL cholesterol. Previously, we were told that saturated fats are considered to be the "bad fats" and they have the opposite effect of raising cholesterol. However, it is very interesting to note that ongoing research may now be suggesting that the saturated fats may not be all that bad for you, after all. Keep in mind that the "jury is still out" on saturated fats in your diet and know that dietary fat research is ongoing, as well it should be. Further, recent studies suggest that saturated fats may increase your HDL (good cholesterol).

In my opinion, based on literature review and clinical experience, the negative impact of saturated fats in your diet has been grossly overstated. Further, as I found in my patients, a diet too low in dietary fats may lead to joint pains from a lack of joint lubrication. Because insulin turns on cholesterol production, it is important to realize that refined sugar has a very significant negative impact on your blood cholesterol levels.

This discussion of cholesterol and low fat diets would not be complete without some further information about trans fats in your diet. **So, why all the fuss about trans fats?** It is proven that trans fats tend to raise your bad (LDL) cholesterol levels and lower your good (HDL) cholesterol levels (just like sugar). Therefore, eating significant amounts of trans fats will increase your risk of developing heart disease and stroke, and will also increase your risk of developing Type 2 (adult onset) Diabetes. Wow, this sounds just like the negative consequences of eating refined sugar.

The good news on trans fats is that they are becoming more and more difficult to find. Fortunately, with voluntary and legislative changes, there are fewer and fewer trans fats found in our popular foods. For example, New York City and Philadelphia have essentially banned trans fats. Many fast food restaurants are now, or will be in the near future, "trans fat-free", and it is recommended that you avoid cooking with trans fats at home.

DIETARY FIBER LOWERS CHOLESTEROL

Clearly, refined sugar in the diet has been shown to impact your blood cholesterol levels. In addition to the cholesterol lowering benefits of the SOS Diet, **a high fiber diet has a role in helping to lower cholesterol levels.** So, what is a high fiber diet? A high fiber diet is generally defined as about 30 grams of dietary fiber per day. This increased dietary fiber may also help lower your blood cholesterol levels, by perhaps as much as 10 to 15%. Other benefits of a high fiber diet include decreased risk for colon and rectal cancer, treatment of diarrhea and/or constipation, treatment of Irritable Bowel Syndrome (IBS), and decreased risk of developing diverticulitis if you have diverticulosis. Enough about fiber at this point... there is much more short and simple dietary fiber information for you to review in Chapter 9, "Fiber is Your Friend".

UNDERSTANDING YOUR CHOLESTEROL NUMBERS

Your health care provider will periodically order blood tests to check your cholesterol, often referred to as a "coronary risk panel", or "lipid profile". This test will usually include total cholesterol, HDL and LDL cholesterol, and your triglyceride level. Your HDL cholesterol is thought to protect against heart disease, so this HDL cholesterol is considered to be your "good" cholesterol. Therefore, the higher the HDL level, the better. An HDL level below 40 is undesirable, and an HDL of 60 or greater is considered to offer protection against heart disease. With regard to the risk of heart disease, a total cholesterol number of 200 or less is favorable. Simply stated, your HDL is considered "good" because it transports cholesterol out of the blood stream back to the liver to reduce build-up in the arteries. Your LDL is considered "bad" because it does the opposite by transporting cholesterol from the liver to the blood stream where it can increase build-up in the arteries. So, __H__DL = __H__ealthy, and __L__DL = __L__ousy.

You may also see a calculated value, called the total cholesterol/HDL ratio. If you do not have a report of this ratio, you can easily calculate it yourself. The TC/HDL ratio is calculated by merely dividing the total cholesterol number by the HDL number. Although there is not universal agreement, many experts believe that this total cholesterol/HDL ratio (TC/HDL) is more meaningful to predict heart disease than the total cholesterol value alone. This TC/HDL ratio concept makes sense because it gives added weight to the HDL value when assessing these multiple blood cholesterol values for the risk of heart disease. **As a general guideline, a TC/HDL ratio of 4.0 or less is desirable, and this value would indicate low risk for heart disease.**

A triglyceride level of less than 150 is considered desirable, but this number is not as commonly used to predict the risk of heart disease. Elevated triglyceride levels are often seen with excess alcohol use and very high triglyceride levels may cause pancreatitis.

To summarize my opinion regarding dietary impact on cholesterol, refined sugar and trans fats are bad, unsaturated fats are good, and more research is needed to assess whether saturated fats are good or bad. Personally, I do not avoid saturated fats in my own diet, nor do I advise my patients to do so.

CHAPTER 5
BOTTOM LINE TAKE HOME MESSAGE

The majority of your cholesterol is manufactured in your body, and does <u>not</u> come from eating fats or cholesterol. One side effect from refined sugar in your diet is the increased levels of circulating insulin. The circulating insulin then directs the liver to manufacture more cholesterol.

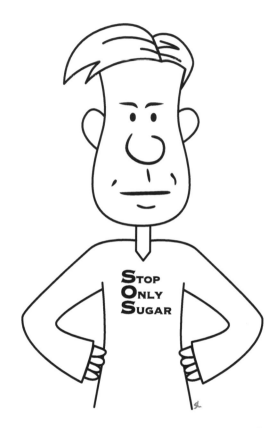

Sugar, you are bad!

CHAPTER 6
SO-CALLED SUGAR "BENEFITS" &
NUMEROUS SUGAR SIDE EFFECTS

Let's pretend for a moment that you and I have just discovered or invented a new food product that we call refined sugar. Before we can take this new product to the general public, we have to obtain the approval of the Food and Drug Administration (FDA). In the United States, new medications and food additives cannot be released to the general public unless they are thoroughly reviewed for safety and approved by this agency of the Federal Government.

So, you have just hired me as your expert Digestive Health Physician "Consultant" to present the refined sugar information to the FDA. What follows is an imaginary example of how this process might work with our presentation of this new food additive product called "refined sugar."

Therefore, we have submitted the following information to the Food and Drug Administration to seek approval to market this refined sugar product to the general public.

Our new product is called "Refined Sugar" (commonly referred to as table sugar). The official chemical name is **Sucrose**. It consists of two equal parts of simple sugars, and this technically makes the product a disaccharide (two sugars). The two simple sugars that make up **Sucrose** are **50% Glucose** and **50% Fructose**.

BENEFITS OF REFINED SUGAR

- It tastes good
- It tastes real good
- Makes you want more and more

PARTIAL LIST OF REPORTED AND POTENTIAL SIDE EFFECTS OF REFINED SUGAR

- Sugar is stored in your body as <u>body fat</u>
- Causes dental cavities
- May lead to childhood obesity
- May lead to adult obesity
- Resulting obesity is a major cause of female infertility
- May lead to childhood Type 2 diabetes
- May lead to adult Type 2 diabetes
- May cause elevated blood cholesterol from excess circulating insulin
- May lead to increased risk for heart attack
- May lead to increased risk for stroke
- May lead to increased risk for vascular disease
- May lead to increased risk for bacterial, viral, and yeast infections
- May cause pancreatic insufficiency
- May suppress the immune system leading to frequent illness
- Obesity leads to increased risk of multiple cancers, including breast, colorectal and others
- Worsens abdominal cramping and bloating symptoms of Irritable Bowel Syndrome (IBS)
- May cause reactive hypoglycemia with mood swings
- May cause hyperactivity in children and others
- May cause addiction to the taste
- Likely will cause a shorter lifespan secondary to the above health risks

At this point in our formal presentation to the FDA, they were probably considering whether or not to throw me out of the 19th story window of the FDA Headquarters Building, or perhaps just to have me admitted for a psychiatric mental status examination...

Obviously, this is a tongue-in-cheek imaginary presentation to the Food and Drug Administration of the United States Federal Government. As one goes back and reviews the list of benefits and the list of potential side effects of refined sugar, one might question whether or not we would get FDA approval. Obviously, this presentation was never given to the Food and Drug Administration. Refined sugar has been with us for many, many years since it was initially imported and is now grown in the United States.

What kind of a trend are we on? In the past decade, consumption of refined sugar in the USA has steadily increased. As noted previously, various studies show the current average consumption of refined sugar in the United States to be about **140 pounds of sugar per person per year**. This means that the USA average refined sugar intake is **about 2 to 3 pounds of sugar per person each and every week**! Wow, no wonder they can't hardly make those cholesterol-lowering and diabetes medications fast enough...

CHAPTER 6
BOTTOM LINE TAKE HOME MESSAGE

Dietary refined sugar, in addition to adding pounds of body fat, also may be a significant factor in raising blood cholesterol levels. As noted above, there are other numerous potential side effects that have a very profound effect on your personal health. All of these side effects are eliminated with the SOS Diet – Stop Only Sugar!

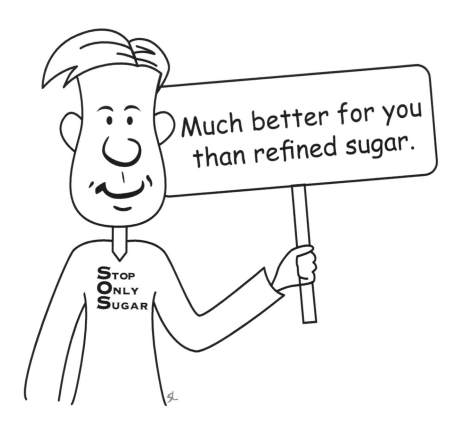

CHAPTER 7
SUGAR SUBSTITUTES... ARE THEY SAFE? — YES, YES, AND MORE YES!

WITHOUT A DOUBT, THEY ARE MUCH BETTER FOR YOU THAN REFINED SUGAR!

As you likely know, you can find almost any information you need on the Internet to give support for or against just about any product, idea, or subject. This, of course, also applies to sugar substitutes. I recommend that you view any and all information found on the Internet with caution and **always consider the source** of the information. This may especially apply to medical advice, and you should always assess whether it is based on science or merely an opinion. Following these simple guidelines, I have included the following information regarding sugar substitutes.

Please note that the sources mentioned are completely credible and offer valid, proven, and scientific findings regarding sugar substitutes. Please recall that I continue to maintain my fellowship status in both the American College of Surgeons and the American Society of Colon and Rectal Surgeons. I have been practicing colorectal surgery for the past 20 plus years, seeing many thousands of patients, and a large part of my practice is devoted to nutrition, weight management, cancer screening, and overall digestive health. Trust me, this education, training, and clinical experience has made me very skeptical about various medical claims, both good and bad, and I always want to see and assess for myself the true and valid evidence. With this perspective, please review the following information.

There is substantial public domain information regarding sugar substitutes in various publications and on the Internet. There is excellent information also available regarding sugar substitutes from the very reputable and highly respected **Mayo Clinic** and I highly recommend that you visit their website at www.mayoclinic.com.

To begin, let us ask and answer this question... "What are artificial sweeteners?"

Artificial sweeteners are products that offer the taste and sweetness of sugar without the many negative refined sugar side effects. Be aware that the commonly used artificial sweeteners are much sweeter than refined sugar, so it takes a much smaller amount to create the same sweet taste. Further, the products made with the commonly used artificial sweeteners have little to no potential for causing weight gain, along with none of the many other unhealthy side effects of refined sugar. On their website, the Mayo Clinic makes this rather obvious statement. "Artificial sweeteners are often used as part of a weight-loss plan or as a means to control weight gain."

Now for the critical question... "What about the safety of artificial sweeteners?"

Artificial sweeteners are often the subject of stories in the popular press and on the Internet, claiming that they cause a variety of health problems, including cancer. In my opinion, this is completely untrue, has no basis in scientific fact, and I don't believe it for a minute. My opinion is based on scientific studies and the facts, and I will justify my belief and my position below. **According to the National Cancer Institute, there is no scientific evidence that any of the artificial sweeteners approved for use in the United States cause cancer. Further, numerous truly scientific studies confirm that artificial sweeteners are safe for the general population.** Please do yourself a favor and always remain very skeptical and wary of health and illness claims on the Internet. You must always consider the source of such information. Further, always, always look at the real hard scientific evidence regarding the health or illness claims of any product.

The following is from the **U. S. Department of Health and Human Services and the Food and Drug Administration** (2006). I have added my personal opinion and comments to their assessment of sugar substitutes:

Three very commonly used sugar substitutes have been approved by the Food and Drug Administration (FDA), including **saccharin** (Sweet'n Low), **aspartame** (NutraSweet and Equal), and **sucralose** (Splenda), for use in a variety of foods. Let's look at each of these from the standpoint of **true scientific research**, and the "test of time".

<u>SACCHARIN</u> (Sweet'n Low brand, & others) – Believe it or not, this has been around for nearly 130 years! Therefore, the grandparent of all sugar substitutes is saccharin. Discovered in 1878, it was used during both World War I and World War II to sweeten foods, helping to compensate for sugar shortages and rationing. It is **300 times sweeter than sugar**. Now here's some more recent saccharin history. In 1977, a Canadian study looked specifically at the role of impurities and other suspected tumor causes (such as parasites) in test animals. This study showed that extremely high doses of saccharin may cause bladder cancer in rats. However, this study was conducted with **the test rats being fed the equivalent of as many as 800 diet sodas a day**. Hey boys and girls, even I, as one who really enjoys diet soft drinks, don't drink that much diet soda. For consumers who use saccharin, the key to a lower risk may be moderation, as is the case with many foods that can cause problems when eaten in excess. Or, if you wish, just avoid saccharin. In my opinion, along with many other health care professionals, professional societies and associations, the use of saccharin has clearly been shown to be acceptable and safe.

Suffice it to say, saccharin has been around for about 130 years, and in very common use over the past 30 years. Guess what… and this is very important; there has been **no** resulting increase or epidemic of bladder cancer. I believe the take-home message is to use saccharin in moderation, and limit your intake of saccharin-sweetened diet soft drinks to no more than 100 bottles or cans per day. Of course, this is only 1/8 of what was found to cause bladder cancer in some Canadian rats. You know, I believe I can control myself and do this... just kidding, just kidding.

ASPARTAME (NutraSweet, Equal & other brands) - Approved in 1981, aspartame is **180 times sweeter than sugar**. As noted, aspartame is sold under trade names such as NutraSweet and Equal, and **is one of the most thoroughly tested and studied food additives the agency has ever approved**. The FDA has thoroughly reviewed more than 100 toxicological and clinical studies. **This is worth repeating... more than 100 scientific studies confirm the safety of aspartame**! This in-depth review of these many scientific studies confirms over and over again that aspartame is very safe for the general population.

As you may well be aware, multiple Internet websites have screaming headlines and well-written text that attempt to link aspartame consumption to systemic lupus, multiple sclerosis, vision problems, headaches, fatigue, and even Alzheimer's disease. Please be aware that the FDA's Division of Health Effects Evaluation states there is no "credible evidence" to support, for example, a link between aspartame and multiple sclerosis or systemic lupus. It is known that a small number of people do get headaches from aspartame, and if this occurs, then these individuals should certainly avoid aspartame. Regarding headaches, I actually have many more patients report to me that the frequency of their migraine headaches has been significantly decreased since they started the SOS Diet. In support of this, there are also reports in the scientific literature linking refined sugar in the diet to migraine headaches. However, if an individual does experience headaches related to aspartame, then they should certainly avoid aspartame. Further, these individuals still have the option of using Splenda brand or other artificial sweeteners.

You may have heard that aspartame causes an increased sugar craving. In my extensive clinical and personal experience, this is absolutely not true. To support this, there are reports in well respected scientific literature that strongly deny this claim of increased appetite or sugar craving from aspartame. Further, aspartame is proven to be an important part of an effective weight loss program.

You will also find the aspartame-methanol scare all over the Internet as well. Aspartame ingestion does result in the production of methanol, formaldehyde and formate, substances that should be considered toxic, but only at high doses. But the levels formed by aspartame are modest, and substances such as methanol are actually found in higher amounts in common food products such as citrus juices and tomatoes. Methanol is a natural and harmless by-product of the breakdown of many commonly consumed foods. The methanol produced by the metabolism of aspartame is identical to that which is provided in much larger amounts from fruits, vegetables and their juices and is part of the normal diet. In fact, **a cup of tomato juice provides about six times more methanol than a cup of an aspartame-sweetened soft drink**. Regarding aspartame-related methanol production, know that you would have to drink somewhere between 600 and 1700 cans of aspartame-sweetened diet soft drinks at one sitting to cause any methanol toxicity in the human body. Quite unlikely, wouldn't you say?

Aspartame has come under fire in recent years from individuals who have used the Internet in an attempt to link the sweetener to brain tumors and other serious disorders. However, the FDA stands behind its original approval of aspartame, and subsequent evaluations have shown that this product, one of the most thoroughly tested in FDA history, is safe with no evidence of health risk. Bottom line... **there is no credible evidence to support any health risk from aspartame.** As you look at the objective evidence, it is, in my opinion, clearly much safer than the health risks from refined sugar!

SUCRALOSE (Splenda brand) – This is commonly known by its trade name, Splenda. Sucralose tastes like sugar because it is made from table sugar. Splenda is **600 times sweeter than refined sugar**, but it cannot be digested, so it adds no harmful refined sugar or calories to food. Because sucralose is so much sweeter than sugar, it is bulked up with maltodextrin, a starchy powder, so it will measure more like sugar. It has a good shelf life and does not degrade when exposed to heat, so it can also be used for cooking. **Further, numerous studies have shown that Splenda does not affect blood glucose levels, so it is a healthy option for diabetics.**

Now, how on earth did they make Splenda from refined sugar? Basically, they just rearranged a few atoms and atom groups. Technically and chemically speaking, Splenda is manufactured by the selective chlorination of sucrose, in which three of the hydroxyl groups (OH-) are replaced with three chlorine (Cl-) atoms. In simple terms, they took off three (OH-) groups, and replaced them with three (Cl-) atoms. By the way, both the (OH-) group and (Cl-) atom are all "natural" occurring chemical substances found throughout the human body, that you cannot live without. Therefore, as noted on the Splenda packaging, it is actually true that it is, "Made from sugar so it tastes like sugar."

Splenda was first approved for use in Canada in 1991. Subsequent approvals came in Australia in 1993, in New Zealand in 1996, in the United States in 1998, and in the European Union in 2004. As of 2006, it had been approved in over 60 countries, and today Splenda is the leading sugar substitute product based on world-wide sales.

Regarding the safety of Splenda, one report from Australia reviewed two studies on rats that were given very high doses of Splenda and this showed a decrease in the weight of the rat thymus glands. For this to occur in a 150 pound human, one would have to consume more than 17,200 individual Splenda packets every day for approximately one month. This Australian report also showed that the dose required to provoke any immunological response in these rat studies was nearly 4,300 Splenda packets per day. Of course, after evaluation of this data and other toxicological findings, they now report that sucralose (Splenda) does not pose any hazard at all to public health. Further, one research report on Japanese mice showed that DNA damage may occur in the mice if they were given the human equivalent of about 11,450 packets of Splenda per day. So, here's my advice regarding Splenda... try to limit yourself to no more than 3,000 packets per day, just to be safe! I think I can do this!

As mentioned, Splenda is 600 times sweeter than sugar. After **reviewing more than 110 animal and human safety studies conducted over 20 years**, the FDA approved it in 1998 as a tabletop sweetener and for use in products such as baked goods, nonalcoholic beverages, chewing gum, frozen dairy desserts, fruit juices, and gelatins. Then, in 2006, the FDA amended its regulation to allow Splenda (sucralose) as a general-purpose sweetener for all foods. Bottom line... Splenda is a very safe product and much better for you than refined sugar.

STEVIA AS A SUGAR SUBSTITUTE

Stevia is a naturally grown plant and is a member of the sunflower family. It is widely grown for its sweet leaves. Depending on the concentration, which may vary widely, stevia extracts can be prepared to be up to 300 times sweeter than refined sugar. It is in common worldwide use as a sugar substitute. The sweet taste of stevia has a slower onset than sugar, and some report a mild aftertaste, but only in high concentrations. Stevia is becoming more and more popular as a sugar substitute because, like other sugar substitutes, it does not raise blood glucose, and therefore does not cause significant insulin secretion.

Multiple studies have shown no negative effects on general health associated with doses equivalent to a 150 pound person drinking between 1,000 and 2,000 8-ounce servings of a stevia-sweetened beverage. There were no reported effects on any organ, including kidneys, male reproductive organs, reproduction, growth or development of adults or their offspring, no significant blood pressure effects in healthy subjects, and did not affect blood sugar. Further studies reported that consuming 29 packets of stevia sweetener or drinking approximately eight 8-ounce servings of a stevia-sweetened beverage every day for up to 16 weeks had no effect on blood pressure, or on blood sugar control in diabetic test subjects.

Stevia is widely used as a sweetener in Japan, and it is now available in Canada as a dietary supplement. In fact, the Japanese use stevia in many food and drink products, and Japan currently consumes more stevia than any other country, with stevia accounting for 40% of their sweetener market. From a production standpoint, China is the world's largest exporter of stevia.

In the early 1990's, based on their stated inadequate toxicology information and safety reports, the FDA labeled stevia as an "unsafe food additive" and restricted its import. This decision was controversial, and it should be noted that stevia occurs naturally, with no patent required to produce it. However, in 2008, the FDA gave a "no objection" approval for GRAS (generally recognized as safe) status to various commercial sugar substitutes which are created from and wholly derived for the stevia plant. In my opinion, the research and use experience shows stevia to be a very safe sugar substitute, in the same manner as saccharin, aspartame, and sucralose. We will all certainly be seeing more stevia sweetened products in the near future.

SUGAR ALCOHOLS

Many sugar free foods, gum, and beverages today are "sweetened' with a product called sugar alcohols. There are various types of sugar alcohols in use today. Like other sugar substitutes, they taste sweet, but are only partially absorbed by our bodies and therefore, do not have the same effects as refined sugar. Let's take a look at these sugar alcohols.

Four sugar alcohols found in common use today are (1) maltitol, (2) xylitol, (3) sorbitol, and (4) mannitol, and there are others as well. Sugar alcohols are considered to be carbohydrates, but **they are neither sugar nor alcohol**. You cannot become intoxicated or drunk on sugar alcohols since they have no ethanol, which is the alcohol in liquor, wine, and beer. Chemically, they are known as "polyols", and part of their chemical structure is similar to sugar, and part is similar to alcohol, hence the chemical name "sugar alcohols".

These commonly used **sugar alcohols are naturally occurring substances that are found in plants, sugar, and starches.** Recall that they taste sweet, but they are not completely absorbed by the body. Therefore, unlike refined sugar, sugar alcohols are not stored as fat, have much less impact on blood sugar levels, and do not result in elevated blood cholesterol. Further, dental research has shown that sugar alcohols do not promote tooth decay as refined sugars do. In addition to food and beverages, sugar alcohols are often used to sweeten chewing gum. For example, "Extra" brand of sugar free gum contains both sorbitol and mannitol, and these sugar alcohols are identified on the label of these products.

If a product is marketed as sugar free, food manufacturers will show the sugar alcohols as ingredients in their products, usually as a separate line item in the list of ingredients. The names of the individual sugar alcohols will usually also be shown on the ingredient list of any product that contains them. The various sugar alcohols used today have a varying range of sweetness, and in many products you will see a mixture of sugar alcohols used along with the other three common safe sugar substitutes including saccharin, aspartame, or sucralose, as previously reviewed.

Always be aware that any food may cause different reactions and side effects in different people. With regard to the sugar alcohols, some people report a laxative effect, even to the point of abdominal cramping and diarrhea. As with many products, these abdominal symptoms from sugar alcohols now seem to be related to the amount ingested. For example, because of resulting cramps and diarrhea, some people cannot eat sugar free ice cream with sugar alcohols, but they have absolutely no problems with the small amount of sugar alcohols in sugar free gum. In my personal and patient experience, these abdominal symptoms are clearly related to the volume of the sugar alcohols ingested. For example, if you wish to try sugar free ice cream sweetened with sugar alcohols, start with a small serving (perhaps one cup) to see if you may experience any side effects such as cramps and diarrhea. If you experience no side effects, then slowly increase your portion size as desired and tolerated.

In my practice, this is the take-home message that works for me and my patients. With regard to how you individually react to various products, YOU must be your own detective. Whenever you have a reaction to any food, drink, or medication (prescription or over-the-counter) that you have put into your body, it is essential that you recall and review what you have consumed in your diet in the past 12 to 24 hours. For example, if you experience cramps and diarrhea from ingesting sugar free ice cream with the sugar alcohols, or headaches from aspartame, then you should individually avoid these products. However, it is totally inappropriate and just wrong for you, for me, or for others to then believe that all people will react in this same way. Again, **YOU must be your own food detective**, and you will soon learn what does and does not work for you on your way to a much healthier lifestyle without refined sugar on the SOS Diet.

As a medical scientist, please know that I have looked at and will continue to look at these sugar substitute products with a skeptical eye, and I am totally convinced of the safety of all these products. In my opinion, you should be wary of various Internet and other claims about the dangers of sugar substitutes.

Finally, let's keep the good and bad claims in proper perspective. What we are really talking about here is to **avoid all the potential side effects from refined sugar**. For perspective, please compare the various side effects of these sugar substitutes and sugar alcohols to the many side effects of refined sugar (including dental cavities, child and adult diabetes, child and adult obesity, elevated cholesterol, heart disease, risk of stroke, vascular disease, increased risk of various infections, mood swings, hyperactivity, reactive hypoglycemia, obesity-related increased risk of various cancers, along with numerous other refined sugar dangers... whew). In light of this scientific reality, confirmed by the many, many years of safe use of sugar substitutes, **it becomes very clear to me that these sugar substitute products are much better for you than refined sugar!**

Do I personally use artificial sweeteners? You bet I do, and I use them every day. My morning coffee always has sucralose, aspartame, or saccharin (whatever is handy), and my favorite diet soft drink brands are Diet Coke, Diet Mountain Dew, or Coke Zero. I also drink 8 to 10 glasses of water every day. In the evening, to avoid the caffeine, my favorites are any of the Diet Rite brand soft drinks, and the entire Diet Rite product line is caffeine-free, sodium-free and sweetened only with sucralose (Splenda).

CHAPTER 7
BOTTOM LINE TAKE HOME MESSAGE

There is no credible scientific evidence to support many of the claims that the sugar substitutes in widespread use today cause any health problems at all. Based on all the scientific evidence, it is my very strong opinion that the sugar substitutes are much better for you than refined sugar.

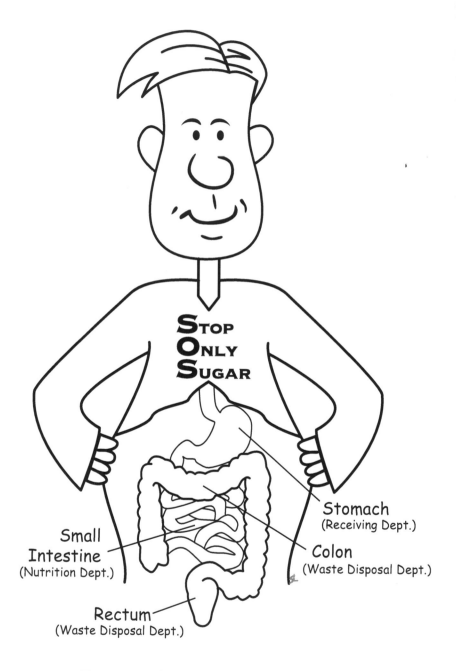

Figure 1 - The Human Digestive System

CHAPTER 8
THE HUMAN DIGESTIVE SYSTEM...
SIMPLIFIED

"THIS IS NOT ROCKET SCIENCE, IT'S JUST DIGESTION."

As you see on the opposite page, a simple diagram of the human digestive system is shown to you by our not-too-shy "Sammy SOS" showing off his own personal internal food processing system.

Before we go any further, let me give you a simple and easy-to-understand way for you to think about your human digestive system. You should think of your digestive system as a very efficient built-in food processing factory that we all carry around in our abdomen, or belly. Think of the human digestive system as this inside-your-body food processing factory with three departments. The first department is the stomach (receiving department). The second department is the small intestine (nutrition department). The third department is the waste disposal system (colon and rectum, or large intestine).

It is important for you to know that your entire digestive system is lined with a very active cell layer called the mucosa. This lining of cells, or mucosa, secretes a thick, clear, slippery substance called mucus. This slippery mucus liquid then serves to lubricate and help food and drink flow through your entire digestive system. Another very important point is that this very active cell layer lining of your digestive system replaces itself about every seven days. What this really means is that **your body gives you a new lining to your colon every week**! Wow, that's impressive, as these cells lining the human digestive system are constantly being shed and being replaced on a daily basis. As you may be thinking, I wonder if this physiologic fact would have any impact on whether the colon is even capable of accumulating pounds of waste and toxins in its wall. Well, I'm glad you just thought of that, and there will be much more on this topic later in Chapter 10 on the absurd and dangerous concept of "Colon Cleansing".

When we eat or drink, the process of digestion begins with the food or drink coming into contact with the saliva in the mouth. Swallowing then occurs and the food or drink passes down the food tube (esophagus) to the stomach (receiving department). The esophagus is really a muscular tube that literally pushes the food or drink from the back of the mouth down into the stomach.

RECEIVING DEPARTMENT (STOMACH)

Once the food or drink arrives in the stomach (receiving department) it is mixed with a potent acid called hydrochloric acid. If one were to take a drop of this acid out of the stomach and put it on your skin, it would literally burn a hole in your skin. However, your stomach has a remarkable ability to resist the effect of this acid which is secreted by cells lining the stomach. Through muscular contractions the food is mixed in the stomach with the stomach acid, and the process of digestion is well on its way. Following a full meal the meal stays in the stomach from about 30 to 60 minutes. Once it is mixed with hydrochloric acid it becomes a thick liquid, which is slowly released into the beginning of the small bowel, called the duodenum, through the pyloric valve. The function of this pyloric valve between the stomach and the duodenum is to allow a proper rate of flow of this semi-solid meal passing from the stomach (receiving department) to the small intestine (nutrition department).

NUTRITION DEPARTMENT (SMALL INTESTINE)

Now that the food or drink we have ingested has left the stomach and entered the beginning of the small intestine (duodenum), the nutrition department of your factory is really going to work. This is where the "action" is, and truly where "digestion" takes place. This small intestine is referred to as "small" because it is a flexible small tube that is only about one inch in diameter. However, it is not small with regard to its length. If removed from the human body, the small intestine would be approximately 22 feet in length. When it is in the human body it is in a constant state of partial muscular contraction, and in your body the small intestine is about 10 feet long. So think of the small intestine in your body as about the size of a one-inch garden hose that is 10 feet long. The reason for this length of small intestine is to provide a very large surface area for contact between the food and the lining of the small intestine where all of our nutrients are absorbed. The length of time it takes for the food and drink to pass through the 10 foot long small intestine usually ranges from about four to twelve hours.

Now, let's take a close-up look at the internal surface area of your nutrition department, or small intestine. If we looked at the lining of the small intestine under a microscope you would see that it had a velvety appearance with many finger-like projections sticking up from the wall of the small intestine. The reason for this is to significantly increase the surface area of the lining of the small intestine to allow for the absorption of the nutrients we have taken into our body. This surface area is greatly increased by the presence of these microscopic finger-like projections. **In fact, if we were to flatten out the total surface of the lining of the small intestine, this surface area would cover the surface of one entire tennis court!** This makes for a very efficient nutrition department that will absorb all of the valuable nutrients that we ingest. During this process, the small intestine is very busy absorbing all of the nutrients that we need to sustain life. This is really the process of our body taking on the fuel that we give it in the form of food and drink. Without your awareness, the small intestine is very busy absorbing the nutrients out of the food and drink we give it such as protein, fats, carbohydrates, vitamins, minerals, and so many other needed nutrients as well. Of interest, only a small portion of the fluid we ingest is absorbed in the small intestine, and by the time the food or drink reaches the end of the small intestine nearly all of the nutrients have been absorbed. This very watery liquid is then passed into the colon and consists of mostly water, waste, and two essential minerals known as electrolytes (sodium and potassium). At the end of the small intestine there is another valve which allows the liquid waste material to slowly leave the end of the small intestine and enter the beginning of the waste disposal department (the large intestine or colon and rectum) in the right lower part of your belly.

WASTE DISPOSAL DEPARTMENT
(COLON AND RECTUM, OR LARGE INTESTINE)

The colon or large intestine now receives this liquid from the small intestine and immediately starts absorbing water, while moving this "waste" out of your body. The colon then passes this liquid waste material up the right side of your belly, across the top of your belly and down the left side of your belly to the rectum where stool is stored until it is appropriate to eliminate the waste material with a bowel movement. In the process of this waste material passing from the beginning of the colon on the right side to the left side and down to the rectum, substantial amounts of water and electrolytes (sodium and potassium) are actively absorbed in the colon. By the time this waste material reaches the lower left side of your belly and goes on down to the rectum in the pelvis, it is much more solid because the water has been absorbed out of the waste material in the process of passing through the colon. The rectum is the lower 10 to 12 inches at the end of your large intestine, where waste is stored until a bowel movement occurs.

It should be noted that the only absolutely essential department of our three department food processing factory is the small intestine, or nutrition department. Humans can live without a stomach, and we can live without a colon and/or rectum. However, the human needs to have at least one-third to one-half of the length of its small intestine so we have the ability to absorb nutrients from the food and drink that we ingest, to sustain life.

Early on in this digestive process, your human digestive system recognizes that you have taken in (ingested) food or drink with sugar. In response to this, your insulin factory (the pancreas, located behind the stomach) receives a signal to release insulin into the first part of the small intestine through a remarkable system of ducts (tubes). In fact, this is the same system of tubes coming down from the liver and gallbladder where bile is also released into the first part of the small intestine to help with the absorption of fats. Unfortunately, with Type 2 diabetes, the insulin factory (pancreas) cannot keep up with the demand due to way too much sugar in the diet, and additional insulin or diabetes medications are needed. Fortunately, many patients with Type 2 diabetes can reduce or eliminate their diabetes medications with an effective weight loss program. Might I suggest the SOS Diet for these patients... you bet I will, and is it ever gratifying for me to share in the weight loss success and subsequent reduction or elimination of the Type 2 diabetes of these many patients and friends.

So there you have a simplified explanation and look at the human digestive system. You have an extremely efficient internal food processing factory to accept food and drink, process it, and get rid of the waste. You don't even have to think about all the great things your internal factory does for you because it is there to serve you. Keep it happy with the SOS Diet, along with fiber and fluids, and it will keep you happy as well. Like I said, "This is not rocket science, it's just digestion."

CHAPTER 8
BOTTOM LINE TAKE HOME MESSAGE

Think of your human digestive system as your personal internal food processing factory with a receiving department (stomach), nutrition department (small intestine), and waste disposal department (colon and rectum). Most of your nutritional needs are absorbed in the small intestine, except for water, sodium and potassium, which are primarily absorbed in the colon. Further, recall that the inner wall of your colon gets a completely new cellular lining (mucosa) each and every week.

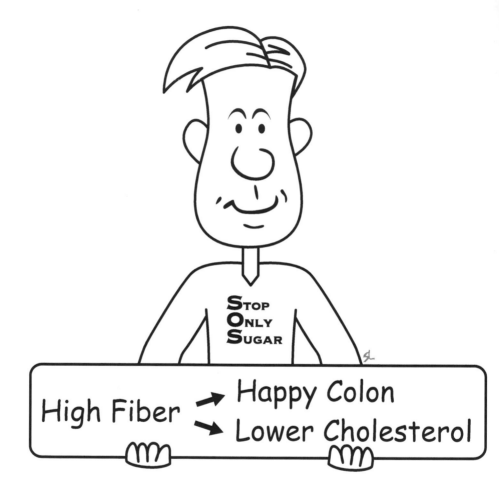

CHAPTER 9
FIBER IS YOUR FRIEND
HIGH FIBER DIETS SIMPLIFIED!

RECALL THE TWO F'S — FIBER AND FLUIDS

Everybody talks about high fiber diets and how many times have you been told to follow a **"High Fiber Diet"**, whatever that is. Unfortunately, many health care professionals and others making these recommendations do not take the time to explain what a high fiber diet truly represents. What follows is a simple straight-forward explanation of high fiber diets and how you can easily make delicious high fiber, low sugar choices. I will also give you a brief summary of the many benefits of increasing the amount of fiber in your diet. Further, know that it is very important that you also pay attention to the amount of fluid in your diet. Unless you are advised otherwise by your health care professional, drink at least six to eight glasses of water each and every day. Also, have a big glass of water with every meal, as this will assist with the process of digestion. So, as you learn these simple guidelines for increasing the amount of fiber in your diet, always recall that the **fiber also needs fluid to work properly in your body.**

There are two terms that you need to know. **Ingestion** is the process of taking the food or drink into your body. **Digestion** is what happens to the food or drink in the human digestive system after you have consumed the food or drink.

Now, this is the only thing you really need to know about fiber in your diet. Fiber is something you ingest that you cannot digest. This **dietary fiber acts like a sponge** to absorb fluid. Like everything else you eat or drink, the fiber in your food or drink first enters the stomach (receiving department), then passes through your small intestine (nutrition department), and enters the colon (waste disposal department). If there is excess fluid in the colon (diarrhea), the fiber absorbs the excess fluid in the colon and slows you down. If there is not enough fluid in the colon (constipation), the fiber absorbs and "hangs on" to the fluid in the food or drink you ingested, and prevents absorption of this fluid into your body. Therefore, because of the way fiber absorbs fluid, fiber will correct both diarrhea and constipation. **Do not ever think of fiber as a laxative, because it is not.** In fact, in my medical practice, I recommend fiber much more for my patients with diarrhea than I do for patients with constipation. Because of the fact that fiber acts like a "sponge" in the colon to absorb fluid, it will readily correct the symptoms of both diarrhea and constipation. So, from this moment on, you should **think of fiber as a "bowel normalizer"** that will correct both diarrhea and/or constipation.

The fact that dietary fiber absorbs liquid gives you another significant benefit. When you ingest the dietary fiber and drink some liquid, the fiber absorbs the liquid while in your stomach, and gives you a "full" feeling. This offers you an almost immediate advantage of decreasing your appetite with almost no additional effort on your part, except to follow the recommended high fiber diet. So, in addition to your dietary fiber acting as a "bowel normalizer", this dietary fiber also serves to decrease your appetite by giving you a full feeling when the fiber absorbs the liquid in your stomach. You may recall this was also confirmed in the medical research I reported to you in Chapter 2.

Further, know that you can also help lower your cholesterol with the addition of dietary fiber. It is believed that by following a high fiber diet with about 30 grams of dietary fiber in one's daily diet may decrease blood cholesterol levels by as much as 10 to 15%. Other benefits of a high fiber diet include decreased risk for colon and rectal cancer, treatment of diarrhea and/or constipation, treatment of Irritable Bowel Syndrome (IBS), and decreased risk of developing diverticulitis if you have diverticulosis. Incidentally, about 60% of adults have diverticulosis, or small pockets on the side of the colon, but most people never have problems and may not even be aware they have diverticulosis (see Appendix D). Finally, please know that if you have diverticulosis, as the majority of adults do, you do NOT have to avoid seeds, nuts, popcorn, peanuts, berries, or any specific foods at all. Just follow a simple high fiber diet.

There are **two types of dietary fiber**, known as **insoluble** and **soluble** fiber. As the names imply, insoluble fiber does not dissolve in water, and soluble fiber does dissolve in water. Wow, that's complicated! Insoluble fiber is found in wheat, rye, bran, many vegetables, and other whole grain products. Soluble fiber is found in oat bran, many fruits, barley, and most legumes (beans).

As mentioned above, **insoluble fiber** means it does not dissolve in water. Another important feature of insoluble fiber is that it cannot be used by the bacteria in your colon as a food source. Therefore, these necessary and beneficial bacteria will not over populate or produce excess intestinal gas.

Soluble fiber, as the name implies, does dissolve in water and forms a thick semi-formed substance in the colon. Soluble fiber also can be metabolized by the bacteria in the colon and, in some people, may temporarily and only briefly increase intestinal gas. Generally, this is not a significant problem, and always lessens over time as your high fiber diet becomes a daily dietary pattern.

Most commercially available fiber supplements, such as Metamucil and Konsyl brands are made from psyllium (pronounced silly-um), which is a naturally occurring high fiber plant that contains both soluble and insoluble fiber. Fiber is very effective in establishing a normal bowel pattern by absorbing fluid, and therefore will help control both diarrhea and constipation. The body cannot absorb either soluble or insoluble fiber, and both types are eventually passed with bowel movements. **You should simply think of a high fiber diet as your bowel normalizer.**

Recall that a simple dietary change of adding about 30 grams of dietary fiber to one's daily diet has many health benefits. In so doing, you will get both soluble and insoluble fiber in your diet. However, don't get hung up in keeping score on your fiber intake and please, do not concern yourself at how much soluble versus insoluble fiber you are getting in your diet. Merely plan to get about **30 grams of total dietary fiber in your diet each and every day**. You will feel better, your bowel function will be better, and this too will help lower your cholesterol. Further, a high fiber diet will help do the following... (1) normalize your bowel pattern by eliminating diarrhea and/ or constipation, (2) prevent diverticulosis from becoming infected leading to diverticulitis, (3) decrease or eliminate abdominal cramps and frequent loose stools due to Irritable Bowel Syndrome (IBS), and (4) will also decrease the risk of developing colorectal cancer.

To briefly summarize Fiber and Fluids: You should have about 30 grams of dietary fiber per day and don't get concerned about whether you are ingesting soluble versus insoluble fiber. Unless you are on a fluid restriction from your health care provider, have at least 6 to 8 glasses of water per day and it is generally a good idea to have a big glass of water with every meal. Unless you enjoy getting up during the night to urinate, you may wish to limit how much water you drink in the evening. Remember that the human body is made up of about 60% water, and we need to replace this water and rehydrate ourselves on a continuing daily basis. We all lose water continuously from the process of just being alive with normal body functions. A guideline I use myself and recommend to my patients is that you are probable adequately hydrated if you feel the urge to urinate during the day about every 2 to 3 hours. Further, your built-in thirst mechanism is very reliable... if you feel thirsty, you are probably dehydrated, and your body is telling you something.

Here are just some brief comments about colon cancer prevention. The bad news is that colon and rectal cancer is the second leading cause of cancer death in the United States today. The good news is that **colon and rectal cancer is almost totally preventable**, so follow the guidelines to have your recommended colonoscopy exam. As recommended by the American Cancer Society: **"Get the test (colonoscopy), Get the polyp, Get the cure."** Also recall that a high fiber diet of about 30 grams of dietary fiber per day will decrease your risk for developing colon and rectal polyps, and therefore decreases the risk for colon and rectal cancer. Please also see Appendix E for specific colorectal cancer screening guidelines.

I continuously have to remind my Cardiology colleagues of my very slanted personal opinion. As a Colorectal Surgeon focused on digestive health, my narrow-minded view is that the major function of the heart is primarily to pump blood to the colon. Of course, when they challenge me on this very biased view, I remind them of the old saying we have all heard about our mothers... "If Mama's not happy, nobody's happy!" As it relates to human digestion, most of us have had personal experiences to support the following... "If the colon's not happy, nobody's happy." My Cardiology colleagues then usually just shake their heads and walk away. I guess they are probably on their way to go out and buy some high fiber, low sugar cereals, breads, or fiber supplements. Makes sense to me...

Remember that "Fiber is your Friend", and know that your new "friend" will permit your fantastic internal food processing system to function properly. Recall that you need about 30 grams of dietary fiber each and every day and remember to drink water with meals and throughout the day. Once you make this high fiber diet and adequate hydration part of your daily dietary routine, you will see and feel the many benefits, and will be strongly motivated to continue. **My final bit of very sincere advice to you is that you take in this recommended 30 grams of daily dietary fiber only on the days you breathe...**

CHAPTER 9
BOTTOM LINE TAKE HOME MESSAGE

You should have about 30 grams of dietary fiber each and every day, and don't concern yourself as to whether it is soluble or insoluble fiber. Drink at least 6 to 8 glasses of water every day, unless you are advised to be on a fluid restriction for some valid medical reason. Think of dietary fiber as your "bowel normalizer".

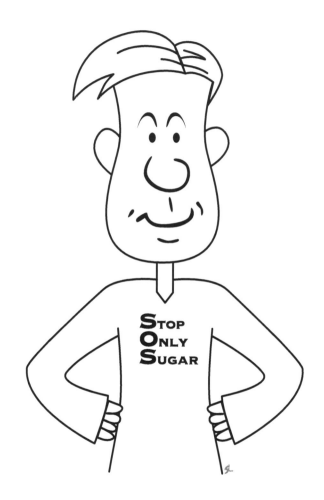

Colon Cleansing . . ?
You gotta be kidding me!

CHAPTER 10
THE MYTH AND DANGERS OF "COLON CLEANSING"

BOTTOM LINE... "DON'T DO IT, AND HERE'S WHY NOT!"

Let me offer you the following opinion regarding the so-called "colon cleansing". Please read this first paragraph very carefully! There is absolutely no way your colon wall is capable of accumulating any toxins or waste. Now, your colon knows this... and I know this... and now, you too will know this.

Hello, people, this is your colon speaking. One more time, for emphasis... there is absolutely no way your colon wall is capable of accumulating any toxins or waste!

I know you are continuously bombarded with all the "colon cleansing" nonsense. They claim you must remove all the evil toxins and waste collected in the wall of your colon, so you can experience a "cleansing of your colon". Then you will magically lose about 5 to 25 pounds almost instantly. Sorry folks, this does not and cannot happen. Your body and your digestive system just does not work this way. The only true weight loss is the loss of body fat. Please keep reading...

KNOW THIS... In fact, colon cleansing actually represents perhaps the most "un-natural" thing you could ever do to your colon. The colon and rectum are referred to as your large intestine, and this organ functions as the "waste disposal system" of your body. Further, the **one and only natural state** of your large intestine is to have stool and bacteria throughout the colon and rectum, and it gets very, very unhappy when it is too clean! Keep reading...

Now, just you wait a minute, Doc! I see on T.V., on the Internet, read the ads, and hear on the radio all these very convincing commercials from many sources. These "colon cleansing" products will clean all these horrible and unhealthy toxins and waste that have accumulated in my colon over the years. Wow, it's amazing that I am still alive and able to move around today with all this collected waste in the wall of my colon. Now, give me a break, Doc, because after I do my colon cleansing I will lose all this weight from the accumulated waste in my body. I will be slim and trim, magically lose my "beer belly", my "love handles" will fall off, and my colon and I will once again become healthy… after I get rid of all that collected waste in the colon wall. Wrong! Keep reading…

To establish some credibility for my opinion on this matter of colon cleansing, let me remind the reader that I completed 14 years of formal medical education, residency, and fellowship training. I am board-certified in Colorectal Surgery, and hold current fellowship status in both the American Society of Colon and Rectal Surgeons (FASCRS) and the American College of Surgeons (FACS). In this regard, I have performed well over 1,000 major surgical procedures on the human colon, held these colons in my surgical hands, viewed them with my own eyes and looked at them under the microscope. Further, I have successfully treated many thousands of additional patients for digestive and nutritional health issues and digestive problems. A partial list of the various digestive illnesses I treat includes Irritable Bowel Syndrome, Intestinal Infections, Colon and Rectal Cancer, Inflammatory Bowel Disease (Proctitis, Ulcerative Colitis, and Crohn's Disease), Diverticulosis and Diverticulitis, Diarrhea, Constipation, common Anorectal Diseases such as hemorrhoids, anal fissures, and many, many others. Further, a large part of my practice is dietary weight management. I will be happy to match my credentials, my experience, and debate any of the other self-proclaimed "experts" in various fields of digestive health, especially as it relates to the accumulation of waste, toxins or really anything in the wall of the human colon.

Now, how can I make such an outrageous claim that disputes all these various T.V., Internet, and radio "experts" that scare you with all their convincing statements about the accumulation of this dangerous waste in your colon? Well, hang on to your seats (so to speak), because **the evidence is very simple, very logical, and will be very convincing... so please, just keep an open mind**. Let's review the following three major points of scientific evidence, (1) you get a new colon lining every week, (2) if you do not have stool and bacteria in your colon, you develop an inflammation in your colon, which is a special kind of colitis, with rectal bleeding and diarrhea, and (3) a too-clean colon may bring on life-threatening infectious colitis, as noted below.

First, let's briefly review the basic digestive system anatomy that you learned in Chapter 8. Recall that your digestive system is essentially a very long muscular "tube" inside your body with various twists and turns and has some wide and some narrow segments along the way from the entry point (mouth) to the exit point (anus). From top to bottom, you will recall that this includes the **stomach** (receiving department), **small intestine** (nutrition department), and the **colon and rectum** (waste disposal department). All of these three "departments" of your digestive system have four layers to their walls. From the inside out, the official anatomic names are the Mucosa, Submucosa, Muscularis, and Serosa (MSMS). Sorry about the boring anatomy lesson, but now, let's get to the scientific facts. For now, just focus on the inner lining of the human colon, called the mucosa. Think of this inner lining (mucosa) of the colon in the same way that you would visualize a lining in the sleeve of your jacket.

Here is a **very, very important scientific fact about the lining of your colon** called the mucosa. Since it is so busy being your waste disposal department, the lining of your colon is one of the most active cellular parts of your body. In fact, **the inner lining or your colon replaces itself about once a week** by shedding cells and growing new ones. This lining (mucosa) is the part of the colon that actively absorbs water and electrolytes (mostly sodium and potassium) as the "waste" material passes through the colon. The water absorption in the colon is a very important function.

> **Now hear this... now hear this... having done surgery on more than 1,000 colons in my career, I have yet to find a colon that has any "toxins" or accumulated waste in it, either to my viewing of the surgical specimen directly during surgery, or when viewing it under the microscope with my consulting pathologist.**

Now what about the dreadful "black-stained" colon you may have heard or read about, seen photos of, or possibly seen on television? Well, now that you are a newly enlightened SOS Diet digestive expert, you know that it is NOT from accumulated toxins in the colon. However, it is from a well documented condition caused by laxative abuse. Yes, you read it right, the colon turns dark brown or black with a condition called "melanosis coli" from the excess use of laxatives made from the senna plant. If you want to get slightly technical, the dark appearance of the colon is caused by pigments taken up by the macrophages in the submucosa (second of the four layers of the colon) and has no great significance except to show visual evidence for chronic laxative abuse.

The senna plant has been used for centuries as a natural laxative by ingesting the leaves or pods of the plant, or by drinking senna tea. It should however, be used as a laxative only on occasion, and not every day. Senna does work well as a laxative, but some people abuse laxatives and their colon may become "lazy" and therefore dependent on these laxatives. Fortunately, this dark appearance of the colon lining from pigmentation of the submucosa is a reversible process which will correct itself over several weeks when the excessive use of senna is stopped. Further, the darkened lining of the colon promptly disappears because you get a whole new lining for your colon every week! This pigmentation has absolutely nothing to do with accumulated toxins in the colon, and is the result of excess use of senna laxatives. Because the lining of the colon replaces itself every week, it is not physically capable of accumulating anything... hey, what a deal, we get a new colon lining every week!

One of my jobs as a colorectal surgeon is to deal with the very serious and life-threatening condition called perforation (hole in the wall) of the colon or rectum, either from trauma, from diverticulitis, from cancer, or from a medical procedure. A perforation can also occur from overly aggressive high pressure enemas to "cleanse" the colon, although this is not common. Now why all this talk about a hole (perforation) in the colon? If a colon perforation is not promptly treated, it is almost always fatal. I mention this to inform you that a colon perforation is almost always treated with repair, along with "diverting, or detouring" the stool away from that portion of the colon that has been injured and then surgically repaired. This colon perforation is nearly always treated with life-saving surgery, and often with placement of a temporary stool diversion bag above the injury site, while the repaired colon beyond this point heals itself.

Now, let's look at what really happens when you have a "super-clean" colon, and therefore, what are the true effects of a genuine "colon cleansing"? Here's where my experience comes in. As a colorectal surgeon, I often have to make a decision to give the patient a temporary stool diversion (a colostomy or ileostomy bag), usually for trauma or disease, so the colon beyond this point can complete the healing process. You may think of this as a temporary "detour" of the stool into a bag above where you want the colon below to have a chance to heal itself. Sorry to bore you with all this, but here's just a bit more technical information. A "stoma" can be located toward the end of the small intestine (ileostomy) or located as part of the colon (colostomy). This "stoma", or opening, is created where the stool comes out into a bag and therefore NO stool or bacteria go into or through the colon beyond the stoma. The stoma is the new end point where the stool and waste material now comes out of the body. It is very important to understand that the colon is still present in the body beyond where the bag is receiving the stool. However, this part of the colon beyond the stoma is super-clean with no bacteria or stool in it, and therefore has truly been "colon cleansed".

Now, what happens to this "cleansed" colon that is now super-clean and has no stool or bacteria? Well, I'm glad you asked… **the**

colon without any stool or any bacteria is now in a very "un-natural" state. This is not at all what it was designed to do, and the colon promptly figures this out. In a short time, this unused segment of colon becomes very inflamed and starts actively bleeding. However, there is no inflammation or bleeding from the upstream colon where the stool is still present. This inflammation and bleeding in the too-clean colon is a well known and described medical condition called "diversion" or "disuse" colitis. Here's a bit more medical jargon... the suffix "itis" on the end of a medical word means inflammation. Therefore, **"colitis"** means inflammation of the colon. In other words, if the colon does NOT have stool and bacteria present, it becomes very inflamed and starts bleeding. **Therefore, a "cleansed colon" is a colon without stool and bacteria and is a very un-natural state that may lead to colitis and bleeding.** Further, the only way to fix this "no stool" colitis (cleansed colon) is to restart the stool going through this segment of colon, and, as if by magic, the colitis (inflammation and bleeding) promptly goes away. So, here's the bottom line... once you get the stool and bacteria back in the colon so it returns to its natural state, all is well within your colon world one more time. Like I said in Chapter 8, "This is not rocket science, it's just digestion."

Another condition that presents with severe diarrhea and significant rectal bleeding is called infectious colitis, or antibiotic-associated colitis. This is yet another example of a "too-clean" colon, where the normal healthy bacteria in the colon have been diminished, usually from taking antibiotics for an infection not related to the colon. For example, a person may have taken these antibiotics for dental work, pneumonia, urinary tract infection, or for many other valid medical reasons. The undesired side effect is that many of the normal and natural bacteria in your colon are also killed off by the properly used antibiotics that were needed to cure an infection somewhere else in your body. However, this uncommon side effect may occur, and a specific type of bacteria that is resistant to the antibiotics now starts to grow in large numbers. If untreated, this may well become life-threatening. This is yet another example of an "un-natural" or "too-clean" environment within the colon with too few of the natural "good guys" type of bacteria. And, guess what, here comes another case of colitis, with severe diarrhea and rectal bleeding, usually due to the overgrowth of bacteria known as Clostridium Difficele. The treatment for this condition is two-fold... one is to give a specific antibiotic to kill off the excess overgrowth of "bad bacteria", and to sometimes replace the good bacteria with foods and supplements such as fresh yogurt, probiotics, and the like.

Well, no wonder your colon will stay so healthy without pouring in all those laxatives and/or doing those dreadful enemas, or doing any "colon cleansing". Now you know that a too-clean colon will only get you and your colon in trouble... possibly serious life-threatening trouble! Now you can say with confidence, "Wow, I feel better already, especially knowing I get a new colon lining every week... what a deal."

Further, now that you will no longer be pouring in all that refined sugar, your colon will really remain healthy, as you stop giving all your friendly colon bacteria all that sugar to work with to make more intestinal gas and cramps. **You know, on the SOS Diet, you may almost be able feel your colon smile... is that possible?**

CHAPTER 10
BOTTOM LINE TAKE HOME MESSAGE

There is no way your colon is capable of accumulating any toxins, or waste in its wall. Colon cleansing is very unnatural and potentially dangerous. Your colon is designed to have stool and bacteria passing through it and it gets very, very unhappy when it is too clean.

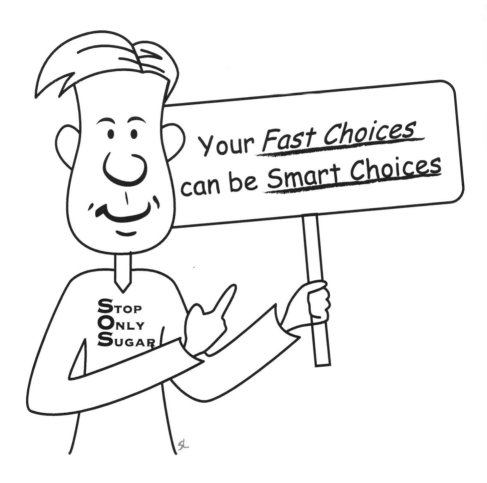

CHAPTER 11
FAST FOOD... FRIEND, FOE, OR MAYBE JUST FAST?

AS ALWAYS, IT'S THE <u>CHOICES</u> YOU MAKE!

Whether or not any food or drink is healthy for you depends on what you choose to consume, and not at all where you choose to consume that food or drink.

As a practicing physician who counsels patients on nutrition and weight management issues on a daily basis, I often hear the comment, "I avoid fast food because it is not good for you." In my opinion, this is a generalization that just is not true, and you must remain aware that **whether or not any meal is "good" for you will depend on your specific food choices, and not necessarily where it was purchased.** What you need to understand about fast food is that it is just that, it is fast!

Why discuss this in a diet book? Since "fast food" is such a significant part of day-to-day life for so many people, let's also make choices to make it as healthy as possible. Like many millions of others, I also eat and enjoy fast food. With the fast food choices I make, it works just fine for me, my weight stays right where I want it, and my cholesterol remains normal. It is common sense that we could all make unhealthy high sugar food choices whether at home, at the finest restaurants, snacking, or eating so-called "fast food". As you will see, **it is all a matter of the "choices" you make.**

With regard to "fast food", or any food we eat for that matter, it must be evaluated in terms of the **choices** we make. Having carefully evaluated their menus and nutritional information, I find very many

healthy choices offered at various "fast food" restaurant chains. Whether or not you choose to eat at "fast food" restaurants is entirely up to you. If you do choose to eat fast food, you will find many healthy, low sugar, high protein, zero trans fat food choices, but you must always focus on the choices you make.

It is very important for you to know that accurate published nutritional information is available from all major fast food establishments. This nutritional information is readily available, upon request, at these fast food restaurants. It is also available on-line. If you have a favorite fast food product that you enjoy, check the sugar content of their nutritional fact sheet, and then make your personal selection based on the lowest sugar content of those items that appeal to you. When at a fast food restaurant, always ask for the **NUTRITION FACT SHEET**, and choose wisely!

It is essential that you always remember that white potatoes (French fries) will be listed as containing no sugar, but recall that potatoes are essentially processed as sugar in the body. In this regard, you should view the carbohydrate content listed for a serving of these potatoes as the sugar content. One large order of French fries may contain as many as 70 grams of sugar... yikes! This same rule applies to corn, as this is also processed as sugar in the body. Further, don't even look at a low fat labels, which are commonly found on the salad dressings, but always check for the amount of sugar. Remember also that just one teaspoon of ketchup has 4 grams of sugar. Get in the habit of thinking SOS - Stop Only Sugar!

Let's review some more information on salads. Salads are great and adding a healthy salad to your meal at a fast food restaurant would be a wise choice. But this salad can turn into an unwise choice if you add a high sugar salad dressing. Most of the sweeter dressings such as "French" or "Russian" dressing and others may contain a large amount of sugar. **In this regard, you must assess the sugar content of the salad dressing and choose only the low sugar content dressings.** Of course, this is true not only when you choose to eat out, but also for salad dressings eaten at your own home or at any restaurant. In my experience, many people are fooled into thinking that a low fat or light salad dressing is always good for them because of the reduced fat content... this may not be true, and you must also assess for high sugar content. As always, remember to read the label for sugar content before using any salad dressing or condiment, and don't fall for the label stating it's low fat, so it must be good for me.

Alright, it's time for lunch, and as usual, we don't have much time, so I pull in to the local **McDonald's Restaurant**. Being the big spender that I am, I'll buy... but let me order for both of us. Well, we now have some food choices to make. My preference would be to order a 5 piece Chicken Selects and this has zero grams of sugar and zero trans fats. To avoid the sugar in the condiments, I would order this meal without any sauce such as the Honey Mustard sauce, Barbecue sauce, Sweet-n-Sour sauce, or ketchup. Wishing to flavor the Chicken Selects with some type of sauce, I would just order this meal with just some plain mustard packets because of my personal preference and taste for mustard. I would order this meal without French fries, and with a large diet soft drink, coffee, or possibly just with water. Let's also have a side salad, but use only the very low sugar content dressing, such as "Newman's Own" Family Recipe Italian Dressing. Way to go, we just had 40 grams of protein, zero trans fats, and only 3 grams of sugar. Now get back to work... you've had your usual 14 minutes for lunch!

Now, let's jump to next week and you and I are going to lunch at the local **Subway Restaurant**. Let's order the following and see how it works out on the SOS Diet. You decide to have a healthy Black Forest Ham on Flat Bread and a large 21 ounce diet/unsweetened tea to have a good amount of healthy fluid with your lunch. Hey, you did great... you just had 3 grams of dietary fiber, only 4 grams of sugar, and a whopping 18 grams of healthy protein, along with some good fluid with your sandwich. And you are full and satisfied. So I decide to have 6 inch Turkey Breast Sandwich on 9 grain bread with a large diet soda. I just had 8 grams of dietary fiber, 4 grams of sugar, and I also get 18 grams of high quality healthy protein. Wow, what a healthy "fast food" lunch we just had.

Next time, we stop at a **Burger King Restaurant** for some of their high quality and tasty Chicken Tenders. I ordered the 8 piece Chicken Tenders with Buffalo Dipping Sauce and a side salad with Ken's Ranch Dressing, along with a large diet soft drink. I was quite hungry so I also had a small order of onion rings. With this filling healthy meal I just had 26 grams of protein, 4 grams of dietary fiber, and only 6 grams of sugar. And I am full and very satisfied.

For a slight change of pace, let's make a stop at **Taco Bell** for some of their great healthy fast food. How about a Grilled Stuft Chicken Burrito, a side order of Mexican Rice, and a couple of glasses of water or a large diet soft drink. Here is our SOS Diet total from this meal at Taco Bell: 35 grams of protein, 8 grams of dietary fiber, and only 6 grams of sugar. Further, know that this great high protein, high fiber meal is not only satisfying when you eat it, but it will also curb your hunger for some time with the added fiber and fluid.

O.K., so now you want to go to **Wendy's**... no problem, and you say you are really hungry. Let's order the following SOS Diet friend-ly meal. You start with a Chicken Caesar Salad, have a small bowl of Wendy's Chili, and top this off with a 5 piece order of Chicken Nuggets with Heartland Ranch Dipping Sauce. Don't forget to have a large soft drink or a few glasses of water, as this will help the fiber work properly. Well, now that your appetite is completely satisfied, here's your nutrition summary: 54 grams of protein, 8 grams of di-etary fiber, and only 9 grams of sugar... good job!

So, please keep the concept of the so-called "fast food" restaurant in proper perspective. Like nearly every other aspect of living your "dietary life", the results of your personal dietary pattern will be a consequence of your **choices**. There are many great fast food choices and if you choose properly, you will continue to enjoy the benefits of following the SOS Diet. **Choose wisely, and enjoy.**

"Fast Food" websites for Nutrition Information

www.McDonalds.com - McDonald's
www.subway.com - Subway
www.bk.com - Burger King
www.tacobell.com - Taco Bell
www.wendys.com - Wendy's

Chapter 11
Bottom Line Take Home Message

Fast food is just that, it is fast. Whether any "fast food" is good or bad for you depends on the choices you make. Always ask for and check the nutrition information sheet readily available at the major fast food restaurants. Simply choose the lowest sugar foods. You will find many healthy choices are available.

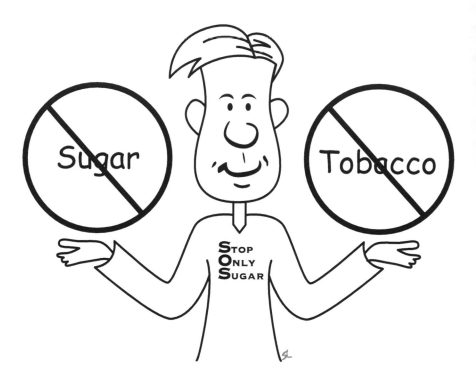

CHAPTER 12
TWO GREAT HEALTHY CHOICES TO HELP AVOID CANCER

(1) SOS DIET AND (2) AVOID ALL TOBACCO

Right now you are probably asking, "Why is my new favorite colorectal surgeon including a chapter on cancer prevention in this short and simple SOS Diet book?"

Good question... and here's the answer. The incidence of various common cancers, including the all-too-common breast and colorectal cancers, is increased with obesity, and is therefore somewhat dietary related. Further, and without question, **the worst non-dietary choice a person can make to ruin their long-term health is to smoke tobacco, which I prefer to call tobacco abuse.** This is followed closely by allowing yourself to be exposed to second-hand smoke, either in your home, car, workplace, or being around smoking friends and others. Further, chewing tobacco also carries significant long-term negative health consequences. So, as you become so much healthier on the SOS Diet with your dietary choices, don't ruin your long-term health with a terrible non-dietary lifestyle choice to smoke cigarettes or to allow yourself to be around second-hand smoke.

Hey, I am just trying to help you become as healthy as you can be. Bear with me as I enlighten you further on the cancer risk reduction by getting down to and maintaining your normal weight with the SOS Diet. Further, by not personally using tobacco and avoiding second-hand smoke, you will substantially reduce your risk for many, many other cancers.

OBESITY AND CANCER

The most commonly used method to determine overweight or obesity is to measure a person's "Body Mass Index", or BMI. The BMI is determined by using weight and height to calculate this BMI number. The BMI is used because, for most people, it correlates with their amount of body fat. An adult who has a BMI between 25 and 29.9 is considered **overweight**. An adult who has a BMI of 30 or higher is considered **obese**. For further details on this BMI calculation, check out the following website: www.cdc.gov/obesity.

Unfortunately, the current statistics from the Centers for Disease Control and Prevention (CDC) show the following. In the USA, 66% of adults aged 20 and older and 32% of children and adolescents aged 2 through 19 years are considered overweight or obese. Further, it has long been known that a high percent of overweight and obese children will carry this medical problem into adulthood. **If you are obese, your predicted life expectancy is decreased by 7 years, and if overweight, life expectancy is decreased by 3 years.**

You may recall that I previously stated that obesity and being overweight have now been proven to significantly increase a person's risk for developing various cancers. Let's look at this from a cancer prevention viewpoint. It has been recently reported in scientific journals that the risk for both breast cancer and colorectal cancer is greatly decreased in patients who have successfully undergone bariatric surgery for their obesity. In fact, in female patients who have returned their weight to normal following this surgery, their risk for breast cancer decreases by an astounding 85%! In both female and male post-bariatric surgery patients, the risk for developing colorectal cancer is decreased by an amazing 70%! There is no longer any debate regarding obesity leading to significantly increased risk for various cancers. This dramatic cancer reduction risk after bariatric surgery is likely due to an improved immune system with elimination of the obesity, and we will all learn more with the ongoing research.

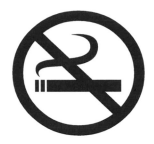

TOBACCO ABUSE AND CANCER

So what else can one do to stay healthy and avoid cancer? **Know this... the single worst choice any person can make to ruin their long-term health is to smoke, and overall, the life expectancy of a smoker is 14 years less than that of a non-smoker!** This means that the overall predicted male life expectancy drops from 75 years to 61 years! Now, let's take a look at the true cancer risk not only from personal tobacco abuse, but also take a closer look at the substantial heath risk from second-hand smoke.

Nobody would argue that smoking causes lung cancer, which is a very serious diagnosis that most often leads to a tragic outcome. The average five year survival after a diagnosis of lung cancer is about 11%, meaning about 89% of people diagnosed with lung cancer are dead within five years. Lung cancer is by far the most common cause of cancer death in the United States. You also need to know that personal tobacco abuse and second-hand smoke significantly increases the risk for many other human cancers. For example, smoking increases the risk of developing colorectal polyps and cancer by about 30%. Further, KNOW THIS... smokers have a significantly increased risk for the following cancers: mouth, throat, larynx (voice box), esophagus, stomach, colon and rectum, bladder, uterus, ovarian, pancreas, prostate, breast, and others. Here's an example... **it is now known that about 40% of bladder cancer is caused from smoking.**

Now, why do smokers (tobacco abusers) get all these cancers? Well, the answer is fairly simple and logical. Smoking and tobacco abuse significantly suppresses the human immune system, and your personal immune system is your first line of defense against many illnesses, including cancer. So, smokers not only get more infections such as colds, flu, and pneumonia, they also have an increased incidence of multiple cancers. This is due to the significant negative impact that smoking has on your immune system. If we could just tune in to what a smoker's immune system would be saying inside our body, it would go something like this. "Here we go again, I just got rid of that cloud of poison from that last cigarette, and now I can't even see to get rid of all this built-up poison and cancer-causing junk that we have been accumulating all these years. If just given the chance, I could have this whole mess cleaned up in just weeks to months, and we'd get back to normal breathing and ability to walk and exercise!"

I previously mentioned **second-hand smoke**, and this is getting more and more negative press every day, as well it should. For example, the latest information shows that **if a person works an eight hour shift in a smoking-allowed work environment (usually a bar or restaurant), this is the equivalent of that worker smoking 1 to 2 packs per day!** Wow, that would be a great place to work with a healthy job-related benefit like that! Many states have now banned smoking in public places, but there is still a long way to go. If your State does not ban smoking in public places, please contact your State legislators to strongly encourage them to pass legislation to ban smoking in all enclosed public places.

The vast majority of heart attacks and vascular disease are from tobacco abuse. The following facts really put this tobacco smoke danger to your heart into proper perspective. In just 3 short years following a city-wide ban of workplace smoking in Pueblo, Colorado, there was an amazing 41 percent reduction in heart attack hospitalizations. Recent CDC statistics show that **second-hand smoke** causes an estimated 46,000 heart disease deaths and 3,000 lung cancer deaths among nonsmokers each year. This same dangerous second-hand smoke health risk occurs if you are a non-smoker and other family members smoke in your presence in the home, car, or other places.

It should absolutely go without saying that parents and other adults should never, ever smoke around children.

But wait a minute, Doc... I have been smoking for years and it won't help me if I quit now, will it? Yes, yes, and more yes! Here's some information you need to know about the many benefits that occur almost immediately and over the course of one year when you quit smoking.

➢ **WITHIN 20 MINUTES** after your last cigarette, your blood pressure and pulse will drop to your normal level and the cooler temperature of your hands and feet will increase to your normal temperature. This is because every cigarette does this: tobacco smoke → constriction (tightening down) of your blood vessels → less blood and oxygen flowing throughout your body → increased blood pressure and pulse to compensate for the decreased blood flow → dramatic increase in heart attacks and vascular disease with continued smoking. Of course, we now know that this also applies to second-hand smoke.

➢ **WITHIN 8 HOURS** after your last cigarette, the carbon monoxide will be out of your bloodstream. In other words, if you smoke a cigarette as infrequently as every 8 hours, you never, ever clear the carbon monoxide out of your blood. You wouldn't consider going out in your driveway and sucking on the tailpipe of your running automobile, would you? Well, that's what you are doing with every cigarette. Most smokers never clear this smoke-related carbon monoxide, as they usually smoke much more than one cigarette every 8 hours.

➢ **WITHIN 24 HOURS** of not smoking your personal risk for a heart attack is decreased.

➢ **WITHIN 48 HOURS** walking becomes easier, your small nerve endings start to grow and repair themselves, and your ability to smell and taste returns to normal, and now all those healthy items on the SOS Diet "Shopping List" will taste even better.

➢ **WITHIN 2 WEEKS TO 3 MONTHS** your lung function improves up to 30% and your overall blood circulation continues to improve.

➤ **WITHIN 1 TO 9 MONTHS** you will experience fewer colds, flu, respiratory infections, coughing, sinus congestion, fatigue and shortness of breath, all due to your healthier lungs and renewed ability to fight infection and handle normal lung mucus and secretions.

➤ **WITHIN 1 YEAR** your risk for a heart attack is now half that of a smoker, and your overall risk for various types of cancers is dramatically reduced.

Be aware that many tobacco abusers require oxygen on a daily basis due to their significant lung damage from smoking. They may require taking their oxygen tank and plastic nasal oxygen hose with them wherever they go and also may have to sleep with it. In effect, they only have a very small portion of their lung function remaining from the damage done to their lungs over the years. Further, know that every person who smokes will ultimately be affected in this way, if they happen to live long enough. The lung may be thought of as a balloon that expands when you inhale and collapses when you exhale. The chronic lung damage from smoking makes the lung much less elastic, so it essentially becomes stretched out and cannot squeeze down. As a result of this non-elastic smoker's lung, the chronic shortness of breath is just like you are drowning and fighting for each breath of air each and every day of your life... clearly not much fun to live this way.

I would not be true to my chosen profession of medicine and this discussion of cancer prevention if I did not mention what I call the "Big Four". The "Big Four" are the four most common potentially life-threatening cancers found in the United States today: 1) breast cancer, 2) prostate cancer, 3) lung cancer, and 4) colorectal cancer. These first two common cancers, breast and prostate, are best treated by early detection and treatment, as modern medicine does not yet know how to prevent them. **For breast cancer, self and professional breast examinations, along with mammograms, are essential for early detection. For the early detection of prostate cancer, professional examination along with prostate specific antigen (PSA) blood testing are essential.** The other two most common cancers, lung and colorectal, are nearly totally preventable with just two words. **For lung cancer prevention – "<u>Don't Smoke</u>" (or be around second-hand smoke), and for colorectal cancer prevention – "<u>Get Checked</u>" (have a colonoscopy).** Further, it is indeed a very sad and telling statistic that shows that, by a wide margin, the number one cancer killer in the USA is lung cancer and number two is colorectal cancer... the two nearly totally preventable cancers! Let's wake up people... get the recommended mammograms and PSA tests, and "Don't Smoke" and "Get Checked" so you do not become one of these cancer death statistics.

One last word on tobacco abuse. If you personally smoke, you must do whatever it takes to quit, and don't ever smoke around non-smokers. Talk to your personal health care provider and know there are many options available to help you quit. Ultimately however, you must make the decision to quit. If you won't quit for yourself, do it for your loved ones... your spouse, your kids, your grandkids, your special someone, or your pet, but just do it.

Please also see Appendix F (When Smokers Quit) for a simple way to help program your subconscious mind to help you quit smoking... I have had hundreds of patients quit using this simple and effective stop smoking technique. YOU can do it too.

CHAPTER 12
BOTTOM LINE TAKE HOME MESSAGE

Make the healthy simple dietary lifestyle **choice** to follow the SOS Diet to drop your unwanted pounds, lower your cholesterol and avoid the increased cancer risks of obesity. If you smoke, or are continuously exposed to second-hand smoke, you must also make the **choice** to personally quit smoking and/or avoid second-hand smoke to become tobacco-free. Also, be sure to follow the recommended guidelines for screening for breast, prostate and colorectal cancer.

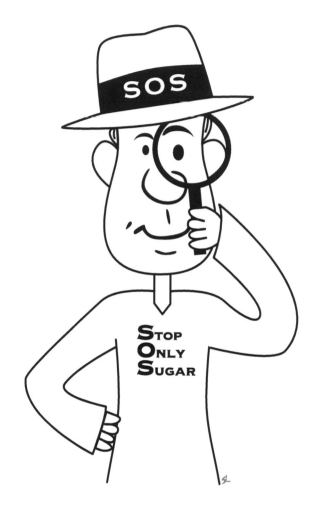

Become a
"Label Reading Detective"

CHAPTER 13
JOIN THE "SUGAR POLICE"

YOU TOO WILL SOON BECOME A
"LABEL READING DETECTIVE"

By now you are probably getting sick and tired of reading my over and over emphasis on how important it is for you to "Become a label reader!" I realize that I have been harping on this throughout this book, but for good reason. I cannot emphasize how very important it is for you to become an informed label reader. Please understand that much of the front side flashy and easily readable printing on food and drink wrapping and packaging is designed to get your attention, and is essentially saying, "Buy me... Buy me!" Certainly some of this is very good information, but know that the writing on the front of the package may or may not give you any valid information about the health benefits or risks of the product. Always read the label for sugar and dietary fiber content and account for the serving size listed on the label.

In my humble opinion, as your new-found diet, nutritional, and label-reading counselor, the most glaring example of what I consider to be very misleading labeling is the low fat or reduced fat labeling on so many food and drink products today. Perhaps the worst example of a label you should absolutely ignore is the "low or reduced fat labels" found even on many candy bars. Oh, that makes it healthy and nutritious for you... please, give me a break! For the most part, I recommend you just disregard these labels because of the near-total ineffectiveness of low fat diets to help people lose weight or lower their cholesterol levels. Please know that your number one priority when reading labels is to check for the grams of sugar content (or carbohydrate content for potato chips, corn chips and various beers), and then also check for the grams of dietary fiber.

Always remember the motto of the "Sugar Police"

LOWEST SUGAR AND HIGHEST FIBER

In this regard, I recently gave a talk on "Healthy Lifestyle Choices" to about 150 adults at a conference in Michigan's beautiful Upper Peninsula. I nearly always do these talks with lots of audience participation and interaction with my "Power Point" slide show. When discussing diets, I asked the audience how many of them tried a low fat diet... about half the audience raised their hands. I then asked how many of them had lost weight and all but one hand went down. When asked how many lowered their cholesterol, if that was a goal of their low fat diet, that single hand went down as well. I was not surprised.

Next, I gave the audience a brief review and a handout going over the basics of the SOS Diet, and the "MISS" (Make It Short & Simple) concept. I suggested to the audience that the problem with nearly all of the diet programs today is that they are just too complicated, they have way too many rules, and they are too difficult, if not impossible, to follow for any length of time. They almost broke out into a cheer over my "Diets are my way too complicated..." comment. At this point one lady raised her hand and stated, "For the first time in my life, I think you have given me a simple diet that I finally understand and know I can follow. I will never eat or drink anything again unless I read the label for the sugar content... this is just too easy!" Wow, I could not have said it better myself. She really did grasp my "MISS" concept – Make It Short & Simple.

As I was leaving the hospital recently, I ran into a colleague who had previously started the SOS Diet. He told me he was experiencing about 7 to 8 pounds a month of weight loss, and he volunteered this comment, "This is so simple, and I don't even know I am on a diet." I then took this opportunity to ask him about his thoughts about label reading for sugar and fiber content with regard to his being on the SOS Diet. He almost looked surprised that I would even ask. He informed me that after our brief initial visit to review the SOS Diet, he really focused on being aware of the sugar and dietary fiber content in the food and drink that he was consuming. He simply said that after a few weeks, he really knew how to avoid the high sugar items, which he did not miss, and he also found it very easy to have about 30 grams of dietary fiber per day. **Like so many others, he became an avid label reader and made a simple lifestyle change.** We agreed that it was very obvious to both of us that he will soon be at his ideal weight and will never have a weight problem again. His current weight loss is 54 pounds in 7 months.

LABEL READING FOR SUGAR & FIBER CONTENT

Always remember that you are reading the nutrition information label for (1) sugar content and (2) dietary fiber content. Further, always be certain to check "serving size" as the sugar and dietary fiber are nearly always listed as "amount per serving". Generally, all you have to do is turn over the package, carton, bottle or can to the label side and just read the label. Sugar and dietary fiber content will nearly always be listed as a separate line item and will be listed in grams. However, for fruits and vegetables that you may purchase individually, or pick them separately and put them in a twist-top bag, you will not find a label listing the sugar content. In prepackaged fruits and vegetables, either fresh or frozen, you will almost always find a label and will find a listing of the grams of sugar, along with the grams of dietary fiber.

Nutrition Facts

Serving Size 1 muffin (57g)
Servings Per Container 6

Amount Per Serving	
Calories 100	Calories from Fat 10
	%Daily Value*
Total Fat 1g	2%
Saturated Fat 0g	15%
Trans Fat 0g	
Polyunsaturated Fat 0g	
Monounsaturated Fat 0g	
Cholest___ 0mg	0%
S___	8%
__al Carbohydra__ 24g	8%
Dietary Fiber 8g	32%
Sugars less than 1g	
Protein 5g	
___in A 0 %	Vitam___
Calc___	Iron 6%

Label from Thomas' Light Muffins

Nearly all fresh fruits and vegetables are good on the SOS Diet, as noted in various other locations throughout this book, so don't concern yourself over the sugar content with these very healthy items. Of course, they contain natural and not refined sugar. However, you need to be careful to note the high sugar content with certain canned fruits, such as fruit cocktail, applesauce and others. Simply check the label on canned fruit items very carefully for the sugar content. By now you have learned that my personal favorite fruit is apples. It really will satisfy your sweet tooth cravings, and you get an extra nutrition bonus from the fiber content. As a snack or dessert, I wash an apple and cut it into slices with an apple slicer. The EKCO brand apple slicer works great for me. Don't peel the apples as the skin is very good for you as well. Apples are a great snack with a few slices of your favorite cheese. I really like Swiss, Cheddar, or Colby cheeses, but add whatever you like that may appeal to your personal taste buds.

Ten further examples of tasty "SOS Diet-friendly" foods for snacks or meals are noted below. The grams of sugar and dietary fiber are taken directly from their package labels and are noted for your quick and easy reference... and this is just what you will now do as a **"Label Reading Detective"**.

10 EXAMPLES OF LABEL INFORMATION ON GREAT FOODS WITH LOW SUGAR , HIGH DIETARY FIBER CONTENT

1) **Original Fiber One brand Cereal** – zero grams sugar & 14 grams fiber per ½ cup serving

2) **Planters brand Dry Roasted Peanuts** – 2 grams sugar & 2 grams dietary fiber per 40 peanut serving - (Hey, mix up some simple SOS Trail Mix – 3 parts Planters dry roasted peanuts & 1 part Original Fiber One cereal... you'll love it!)

3) **Thomas' brand Light Muffins** – 1 gram sugar & 8 grams fiber per muffin (See actual label on the previous page)

4) **Thomas' brand 100 Calorie Bagels** – 1 gram sugar & 4 grams fiber per bagel

5) Brownberry brand Carb Counting Bread – zero grams sugar & 6 grams fiber per 2 slices

6) Sara Lee brand Low Calorie Bread – 2 grams sugar & 5 grams fiber per 2 slices

7) Jif or Skippy brand Peanut Butter – 3 grams sugar & 2 grams fiber per 2 tablespoons

8) Emerald brand Cocoa Roast Almonds – 1 gram sugar & 3 grams dietary fiber per 20 almond serving

9) Triscuit brand Original Crackers – zero grams sugar & 3 grams fiber per serving

10) Wheat Thins brand Fiber Selects Crackers – 4 grams sugar & 5 grams fiber per 13 cracker serving

In closing, let me issue the following "Official SOS Diet Proclamation". By now having completed this brief chapter, I send you my personal congratulations. You have now been accepted into the "Sugar Police Force", and have already been promoted to full "Label Reading Detective" status, with all associated SOS Diet rights and responsibilities. **Never forget our "Sugar Police Motto"** . . .

LOWEST SUGAR AND HIGHEST FIBER

CHAPTER 13
BOTTOM LINE TAKE HOME MESSAGE

You must become an informed and dedicated label reader. Be certain to check your various foods and drink for grams of sugar and grams of dietary fiber and make informed choices of what you decide to eat and drink. In a very short time, you won't even believe you are "on a diet", because you are now making healthy choices that will easily get rid of the excess pounds and may help lower your cholesterol as well.

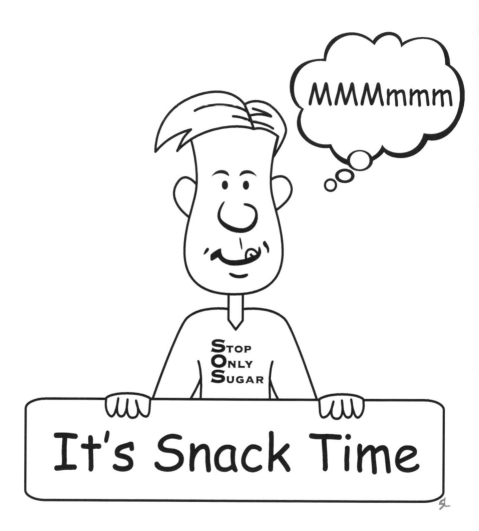

CHAPTER 14
SATISFY YOUR NEED TO SNACK...
WITHOUT THE POUNDS!

KEEP YOUR SWEET TOOTH HAPPY
WITHOUT THE REFINED SUGAR

I must tell you that my sweet tooth is every bit as demanding as your sweet tooth, or worse. We all enjoy the sweet "treats" perhaps because we all grew up drinking the sugar-loaded soft drinks and eating popsicles and candy bars. Of course they came to be known as "treats" and this carried over into what I call the "dessert dilemma". This dilemma is the problem of frequently being offered a dessert after meals when most of us are already too full to eat anything else, but often we are unable to resist the very high sugar ice cream, cake, pie, cheese cake, hot fudge sundae, or the like.

Is this "dessert dilemma" still part of your dietary lifestyle? Unfortunately, these high refined sugar "treats" are all too common, and they just get stored as body fat. Let me be so bold as to suggest to you that there are dessert and snack alternatives that you will find every bit as satisfying, if not more so. Once you learn the simple guidelines of the SOS Diet, you will be able to make dessert choices that you find tasty and filling. Of course, it will be okay to enjoy these desserts and other "treats" on an occasional basis. Hey, we all have to fall off the SOS wagon once in a while... now don't tell anybody, but when I'm out at the local Friday night fish fry, I enjoy a plate of French fries with my delicious deep fried perch dinner. In the warm weather, I may even occasionally have some real ice cream, if sugar free is not available. However, don't you ever tell anybody about this; it is our little secret... and remember, as a Colorectal Surgeon, I have instruments you really do not want to know about!

So what are some other alternatives to satisfying your sweet tooth without ingesting a large amount of sugar? Let's take a typical evening where an individual who happens to be a "snacker", like I am, who may have previously had an enjoyable healthy low refined sugar dinner, but now is having some cravings for a snack. What I have learned to do under these circumstances is to make one or two pieces of toast with high fiber, low sugar whole grain bread, lay on the butter or margarine, smear on the Jif brand peanut butter and Smucker's brand Sugar free Strawberry Jam (my favorites). Now let's look at some details of what this healthy "sweet tooth" snack did for you from a nutrition standpoint. First of all, there are zero grams of sugar in the Smucker's brand Sugar Free Strawberry Jam. In the Jif or Skippy brand Peanut Butter, there are only 3 grams of sugar in two tablespoons. This two tablespoon serving is probably more than what you would actually use with whole grain bread for a good old fashioned peanut butter and jelly sandwich or two slices of toast. In the bread, there are usually 2 or 3 grams of fiber per slice and zero to only 2 or 3 grams of sugar as well. Although you did ingest some sugar with this type of snack, you also ingested a good amount of dietary fiber along with perhaps 8 to 10 grams of protein from the peanut butter. This will also be very satisfying as well as very healthy and nutritious.

I have learned to satisfy my personal sweet tooth with apples. In fact, **my SOS Diet "candy bar" is a crunchy apple.** The Honey Crisp apple variety is a rather crunchy variety with a very sweet taste and has become my favorite apple. Many other types of apples are just as satisfying and taste just as sweet... as always, it's your choice. Other apple varieties that I enjoy are Pink Lady, Fuji, Cameo and Gala, or whatever is on sale and looks good. If one does not like apples to be too sweet, a great choice would be Granny Smith apples as this variety is crunchy and has a less sweet taste to it. Further, you must appreciate the fact that apples also contain fiber. Trust me, you will find these apples and other sweet tooth substitutes will allow you and your sweet tooth to be very satisfied. A great snack is to cut up an apple, and dip it in peanut butter.

Let's say that you had a good day with your SOS Diet with a ham and cheese omelet or bacon and egg breakfast with whole grain high fiber toast with butter (or margarine), peanut butter, and sugar free jam or jelly, if desired. For lunch you had a large chef's salad, but you were careful to use only a dressing that was very low in sugar or sugar free (please, just ignore any low fat label on the dressing). For dinner, you had a large serving of beef, chicken, pork, or fish without any high sugar sauces, a generous serving of various types of green vegetables and a tossed salad with vinegar and oil or other low-sugar type dressing. However, your favorite TV show is about to come on and as I do, you are feeling the urge to have a snack.

Prior to your minor lifestyle change with the SOS Diet, under the above circumstances you may have headed to the kitchen, prepared a large bowl of potato chips or corn chips with some sugar-laden chip dip and "munched" your way throughout your favorite TV show. However, now you know that these potato and corn products essentially wind up as sugar and are stored in your body as body fat. So now you choose to avoid this type of high sugar snacking. Let me suggest an alternative. Let's make the same trip back to the kitchen. This time, you reach for the box of 100% Whole Grain or Fiber Selects Wheat Thins. A quick review of the Whole Grain Wheat Thins label will show that 16 of these Wheat Thins brand crackers contain only 3 grams of sugar and give you an additional 2 grams of fiber. If you choose the Fiber Selects Wheat Thins, then a 13 cracker dose contains 4 grams of sugar and 5 grams of dietary fiber. If you chose Triscuit brand crackers, you will get zero grams of sugar. What I do is take the Wheat Thins brand crackers and put peanut butter on each of the crackers and you will find this to be a very satisfying, filling and enjoyable snack. If you use a total of two tablespoons of "Jif" brand peanut butter, which would be more than enough for 16 wheat thins, you will have ingested only 3 additional grams of sugar, and a very healthy 8 grams of high quality protein. If my "sweet tooth" is acting up, as it often does, I may add a dab of Smucker's sugar free strawberry jam with the peanut butter on each cracker, to sweeten things up. The Smucker's is actually a "freebee" with zero grams of sugar. This is what I would consider to be an example of a healthy snack and one that I am sure you will find, as my patients all tell me they do, to be very filling and satisfying. Win Schuler's also makes a tasty soft cheese spread that is very low sugar and goes great on any variety of low sugar crackers.

Let me emphasize once again that you should not focus on carbohydrate grams when following the SOS Diet, as it is NOT a low carb diet... it is a low sugar diet. However, there are a few exceptions to this suggested guideline, where you should check the carb count when you see sugar listed as zero grams, but you know this is on the SOS Diet "NO-NO" list. **As previously reviewed, these few exceptions include potato chip and corn chip snacks, and beers. With these three items, you should check the carbohydrate gram count, and count that as sugar.** With regard to beer, read the label and choose the lowest carbohydrate beer that appeals to your taste and pocketbook. If the beer label does not have the nutrition information (cans usually do, but some bottles do not), then check the carbohydrate content for that brand on-line. Further, you also are now aware that white potatoes and corn turn to sugar in the body, and the potato chips and corn chips nutrition labels will show no sugar, but a large amount of carbohydrates. With both the potato and corn chips, you must count these carbohydrates as sugar... sorry about that. Try substituting dry roasted peanuts... a great tasting healthy snack!

For the most part, what you really need to remember is this: **refined sugar = bad carbohydrates**. Further, be aware that we all need a daily portion of carbohydrates for a satisfying and reasonable balanced diet. In my opinion, the best choice for healthy made-from-grain carbohydrates is to select whole grain or multi-grain products that are high in fiber and low in sugar. However, you must avoid white breads, pastries, donuts, and the like. Remember, "If it's white, it's just not right." Just two great examples of very satisfying and healthy choices of high fiber low sugar bread products are as follows. Along with other whole grain brands, check these products... two slices of **Brownberry Multigrain "Carb Counting" brand bread** has 6 grams of fiber and zero grams of sugar, and 10 grams of protein.

Two slices of **Sara Lee "45 Calorie" Wheat Bread** has only 2 grams of sugar, along with 5 grams of fiber and 6 grams of protein... either would be a very healthy SOS Diet choice. Way to go, Brownberry and Sara Lee – the SOS Diet likes you.

Another great made-from-grain product that you need to be aware of is the **Thomas' brand "Light Multi-grain Muffins."** What a great satisfying and nutritional product this is, that will serve you well for breakfast or for a snack on your SOS Diet! Check this out... each single muffin contains 8 grams of dietary fiber and less than 1 gram of sugar... WOW! This makes for a great breakfast with a toasted muffin with butter or soft margarine, with or without peanut butter, and I tend to also load it up with the Smucker's sugar free strawberry jam. Many other Smucker's sugar free varieties are also available. You're going to love this choice, either for breakfast, or as a TV watching or evening snack. Thomas also offers their 100 calorie plain bagels and each bagel contains 4 grams of dietary fiber and less than 1 gram of sugar... another SOS Diet WOW!

What about popcorn? Well, everybody loves popcorn and I am no exception. However, you will learn from the list of foods to avoid that corn is one of those foods that converts to sugar when digested, but what sane person would recommend a diet program that did not permit you to have some popcorn! Popcorn also does give you some fiber, so the sugar content is a minus, but the fiber is a plus. Try to limit your popcorn ingestion to 1 to 2 times a week, for sure at the movies, or just for fun at home... but not every day. Of course, you can also enjoy your popcorn with butter and salt.

WHAT ABOUT SALT AND SODIUM?

Regarding salt... my personal preference is to use the Morton brand "Lite Salt" which is half sodium chloride and half potassium chloride, and in my opinion, tastes almost exactly like regular table salt. The advantage of this product is that it gives you some potassium and offers a lower amount of sodium for those individuals who have been advised to limit their amount of sodium intake. A few comments follow about sodium.

A dietary sodium restriction is generally suggested only for a patient who is dealing with high blood pressure, medically known as hypertension. Patients with high blood pressure (hypertension) are usually treated with medications to lower their blood pressure and may also be treated with diuretic medications to decrease body fluids. These patients clearly should minimize their dietary sodium intake. **If you have been advised to reduce your sodium intake by your health care professional, you certainly need to follow that advice.** Further, as you have no doubt noticed, we are all bombarded with information about how bad sodium is for you. However, if you do not have high blood pressure, are not taking any blood pressure reducing medications and are not taking diuretic medications to reduce body fluids, it may not be an issue at all. Further, I find it very interesting that various "experts" are now singing the praises of various salts, such as sea salt. **If you have any questions about a personal sodium restriction, be certain to check with your physician. Be sure to follow the advice of your personal health care provider in this regard.**

Also, isn't it strange that nearly all I.V. (intravenous) fluids and medications given in the hospital are given in saline solution... by the way, this is "salt water" that your body needs for normal functioning. Further, realize that we humans are made up of about 60% water, and this is in the form of what is medically called normal saline (0.9% Sodium Chloride), also known as salt water. I wonder... could it possible be that sodium is perhaps not such a bad guy after all?

Now here is a great "store-bought" ready-to-eat snack. I never leave home without my large can (the 3 pound 4 ounce size) of Planter's brand dry roasted peanuts within easy reach of the driver's seat. This is actually a very healthy food, and should not be considered as just a snack. Many other companies also offer dry roasted peanuts and this is a healthy, very satisfying snack. For example, Planter's brand of dry roasted peanuts offers you the following nutrition in one serving size of approximately 40 dry roasted peanuts, or about two generous "handfuls". With this 40 peanut serving, which is quite filling and very satisfying, you will receive 2 grams of dietary fiber, only

2 grams of sugar and 7 grams of quality protein. This can be a very healthy snack which is totally acceptable on the SOS Diet, and is my personal favorite SOS snack. I find it very filling and satisfying, and it is one of the healthiest snacks you can eat.

Again, let me remind you of the healthy and extremely easy to prepare "SOS Trail Mix" that will be very satisfying, is very high in fiber, very low refined sugar, and high protein. Sound too good to be true... well, it's not. Just mix three parts Planters Dry Roasted Peanuts with one part Original Fiber One Cereal (General Mills product). This Original Fiber One Cereal will actually add some sweetness to this trail mix. This "SOS Trail Mix" is very satisfying and needs no refrigeration, so you can take it with you... to work, in the car, to the movies, or wherever. This home-made trail mix makes for a very healthy and satisfying snack with very low sugar and very high fiber. When I want to sweeten it up a bit, I add one cup of "Emerald" brand Cocoa Roast Almonds to the 3 cups of dry roasted peanuts and the 1 cup of Original Fiber One cereal. With this trail mix, I am actually running out of hiding places for this SOS Diet creation in my office...

What about cheeses? I love them, and so does the SOS Diet! This is yet another healthy low refined sugar food and snack that is actually good for you. My favorite cheeses include Colby, Swiss, Cheddar, and others. As you look at the label on most cheeses, you will find that there is little to no refined sugar, and cheese is an excellent source of protein. For example, Colby cheese offers the following nutritional benefits. A one ounce serving of Colby or Cheddar cheese provides 7 grams of protein and zero grams of sugar. One ounce of Swiss cheese gives you 8 grams of protein and zero grams of refined sugar. In addition, cheese can be a good source of dietary calcium. For example, a 1 ounce serving of Swiss cheese has 272 milligrams of calcium and a 1 ounce serving of Cheddar cheese has 204 milligrams of calcium. However, be aware that cheese does not contain any fiber, so you may wish to have your cheese with some apples, Triscuit Crackers or Wheat Thins. Also, most cheese varieties have zero trans fats.

What about pizza? I love pizza, but order thin crust and don't eat the thick crust around the outside edge, and this will minimize your white flour intake. Fortunately, wheat crust pizza is also becoming more available. Otherwise, enjoy your pizza, but as you start on the SOS Diet, limit it to perhaps once a week.

These are but a few examples of the types of snacks that one can enjoy while following the simple SOS Diet. These snack ideas and suggestions permit you to satisfy your sweet tooth and desire to snack, but doing so in a very healthy manner. This SOS Diet will allow you to continue to lose weight or maintain your weight loss and may help keep your cholesterol levels in a normal range. You will come up with your favorite SOS Diet snack and great ideas on your own, now that you understand the short and simple SOS guidelines. When you come up with an SOS Diet snack winner, please share it with me via email at sosdietdoc@gmail.com, so I can pass it along to your fellow pound-dropping SOS Diet colleagues.

Hint: In recipes, replace the refined sugar with an equal amount of Splenda, or you can also use an equal amount of sugar free syrup. Your baked goods will be just as sweet and tasty.

In addition to the many sugar free foods and snacks being offered in retail stores today, there are many websites offering an amazing variety of sugar free items. If you wish to shop on-line, go to "Google" and enter search: **sugar free food** and you will be pleasantly surprised at the many companies offering a wide variety of quality products from which to choose. Happy snacking!

CHAPTER 14
BOTTOM LINE AND TAKE HOME MESSAGE

There are many very healthy SOS Diet friendly snacks and sweet tooth satisfiers available today. With only this minor lifestyle change to avoid refined sugar and your new focus on reading labels for grams of sugar and dietary fiber, you will find many very nutritious snacks to enjoy that are actually good for you... wow, this is a novel concept!

MY FAVORITE SWEET AND SALTY SNACK

Homemade SOS Trail Mix

3 cups of Planters brand Dry Roasted Peanuts

1 cup Original Fiber One brand cereal and

1 cup Emerald brand Cocoa Roast Almonds

(Betcha can't eat just one handful!)

MY FAVORITE SUGAR FREE SNACKS

Reese's Sugar Free Peanut Butter Cups

Russell Stover Sugar Free Pecan Delights

Hershey's Sugar Free Special Dark Chocolates

Dove Sugar Free Silky Smooth Dark Chocolates

Hershey's Sugar Free Milk Chocolates

Russell Stover Sugar Free Chewy Granola Snack Bars

(Now, don't overdo it and eat the whole bag!)

ANOTHER GREAT SNACK IDEA

Apple wedges dipped in Jif Brand Peanut Butter

(Your sweet tooth will love this!)

Note: Please also see Appendix A,
The SOS Diet "Delicious Dozen".

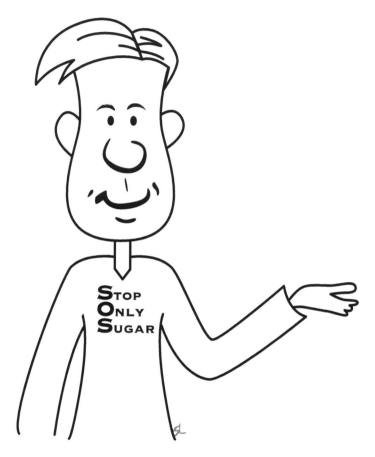

SOS Diet
Myth Busters

CHAPTER 15
TOP TEN SOS DIET MYTH BUSTERS

MYTH # 1. *To be effective, diets have to be complicated, difficult to understand and involve great personal dietary sacrifices.* I hope by now you understand that following the SOS Diet involves only a **minor lifestyle change** to avoid refined sugar. The short and simple SOS Diet will allow you to achieve both early and sustained lifelong weight loss, may help with lowering your cholesterol and will lead to overall better health.

MYTH # 2. *Counting calories is the best way to lose weight.* In my personal and extensive clinical experience with many, many people, this is just too detailed and cumbersome for many of us, myself included. Recall that the concept of the "calorie" was originally used to measure heat output from machines. Don't just look for low calorie labeling. Always check for the sugar content. Focus your personal dietary attention and **label reading for lowest sugar and highest fiber**. Know there are many healthy higher calorie items with very low or zero sugar, contain high quality protein, and these low sugar choices will benefit the new, slimmer and healthier you.

MYTH # 3. *Cholesterol is a very unhealthy substance found in the human body.* If you believe all the hype about how bad cholesterol is, you would want every last drop out of your body! Know this... cholesterol is essential for life. It is found in the cell walls of each and every one of the 50 trillion or so cells in your body and is the building block for steroids, bile, vitamin D, our hormones and **we cannot live without cholesterol**. Elevated blood cholesterol is not healthy, but cholesterol itself is not bad and is necessary to sustain human life.

MYTH # 4. *The fat and cholesterol in your diet are the major causes of elevated cholesterol.* This is not true. Most of your cholesterol (about 85%) is manufactured in your own body, and excess cholesterol may well be triggered by the excess refined sugar in your diet. Two ways to help reduce your cholesterol are to minimize or eliminate refined sugar in your diet and to take in about 30 grams of dietary fiber every day. **Further, it is very important that you always follow your doctor's advice with regard to your cholesterol.**

MYTH # 5. *You must avoid all fat in your diet.* Not true! The current scientific thinking is that you should certainly minimize or eliminate trans fats. There is agreement that unsaturated fats are actually good for you. However, there is disagreement as to whether saturated fats should be avoided. Further, a diet too low in fats may lead to joint pain.

MYTH # 6. *If it is labeled "Low Fat", "Reduced Fat", or "Fat Free", it is always good for you.* Wrong again, sugar breath! Many high sugar food items such as candy bars, salad dressings, jams and jellies, ketchup and other condiments, as well as many other low fat labeled foods are very unhealthy due to the very high sugar content. This sugar will be stored as body fat, add pounds, and likely will increase your cholesterol. Always check the label for the grams of sugar on the label and avoid high sugar items.

MYTH # 7. *Sugar substitutes are not safe.* There is **absolutely no credible evidence** to support these absurd claims. Please review the potential side effects and consequences of refined sugar in your diet… and then never forget how much better the sugar substitutes are for you than refined sugar. Further, there is no credible evidence that sugar substitutes cause any increased sugar cravings at all. Please **critically review the valid scientific research as documented and summarized in Chapter 7.**

MYTH # 8. *Fiber in your diet is a laxative used for constipation.* Nothing could be further from the truth. In my large clinical practice I recommend dietary fiber much more to treat diarrhea than to treat constipation. Understand that fiber is something you ingest (eat or drink) that you cannot digest. It passes through the stomach and small intestine, then goes into the colon and absorbs liquid. It will treat diarrhea or constipation and will decrease pressure in the colon. Dietary fiber should be viewed as a "bowel normalizer". It will also help lower cholesterol, treat Irritable Bowel Syndrome (IBS), prevent diverticulitis and reduce the risk of colon cancer.

MYTH # 9. *Colon cleansing is necessary to clean your colon to lose weight and remove accumulated waste and toxins from your body.* Colon cleansing is actually the most un-natural thing you could ever do to your colon and may lead to potentially very dangerous unintended consequences. It is impossible for your colon wall to accumulate any waste or toxins... please be aware that you get a new lining in your colon every week!

MYTH # 10. *Fast food is bad for you.* Please understand that "fast food" is just that... fast. As with all things in life, every choice we make has consequences. If you choose to eat at "fast food" restaurants, as I often do, choose wisely to avoid the high refined sugar items. Always ask for and check the fast food restaurant **Nutrition Information Fact Sheet** and know that you will find there are many other healthy items on their menus. If they do not offer a nutrition fact sheet, then go somewhere else. Be careful to avoid the many high sugar items and choose from the many low sugar, high protein, zero trans fat items.

CHAPTER 15
BOTTOM LINE TAKE HOME MESSAGE

There are way too many dietary and nutritional "myths" that are too often based on opinion, with absolutely no credible evidence to support them. The SOS Diet is based on research and years of successful clinical experience with real people, just like you. It will offer you early and sustained weight loss. Follow the "MISS" (Make It Short & Simple) concept of the SOS Diet and YOU will be successful... now get out there and SOS - **Stop Only Sugar!**

APPENDIX A – THE SOS DIET "DELICIOUS DOZEN", UM, UM, GOOD... AND GOOD FOR YOU!

1. <u>Planters Dry Roasted Peanuts</u> – Each serving (about 40 peanuts or two good handfuls) contains 2 grams of dietary fiber and 2 grams of sugar... very tasty, filling and healthy. This is a great "take it with you" snack.

2. <u>Original Fiber One Cereal</u> – Original Fiber One Cereal has zero grams of sugar and 14 grams of dietary fiber per half cup serving... Wow! If desired, throw on some fruit, just to add some more healthy and fun taste. Go easy with the milk and recall that a pint (8 ounces) of <u>any</u> milk (skim, reduced fat or whole) contains 12 grams of sugar, or consider using soy milk that contains half the sugar of cow's milk.

3. <u>SOS Trail Mix</u> – Mix 1 cup <u>Original Fiber One Cereal</u> and 3 cups <u>Planters Dry Roasted Peanuts</u>... the Fiber One adds a touch of sweetness... and just like everyone who tries it, you will get hooked on this great tasting and very healthy high fiber snack. This is clearly my personal favorite mixed snack. If I want an extra touch of sweetness, I add some <u>Emerald brand</u> <u>Cocoa Roast Almonds</u>... this offers great taste, very low sugar and very high fiber.

4. <u>Peanut Butter and Sugar Free Jam or Jelly</u> – Use a Thomas' brand "Light" muffin, or Sara Lee brand "45 Calorie", or Brownberry brand Multigrain "Carb Counting", or other high fiber, low sugar whole wheat or whole grain bread. Make yourself some toast, or make a peanut butter and jelly sandwich, using soft margarine, with Jif or Skippy brand peanut butter and Smucker's brand sugar free jam or jelly... this is a great low sugar, high fiber filling snack or light meal.

5. <u>Cheese and Crackers</u> – Swiss, Colby, Cheddar, or your favorite cheese slices on Wheat Thins (I love the Fiber Selects variety), or Triscuit Crackers… this is a great satisfying and filling high protein, high calcium snack. These crackers are also very good with the softer cheese spreads such as Win Schuler's Original Cheddar, or other tasty brands.

6. <u>Sugar free Dark Chocolate</u> - Hershey's brand Sugar free Special Dark Chocolate pieces – and a 5 piece serving has zero grams of sugar and four grams of dietary fiber. "Dove" brand also offers a variety of great tasting sugar free light and dark chocolates. Betcha can't eat just one… but don't eat the whole bag!

7. <u>Apples and Cheese</u> – Cut up a Honey Crisp (sweeter), Granny Smith (less sweet), or your favorite apple and enjoy it with slices of your favorite cheese (I prefer Swiss, Cheddar, or Colby)… and the extra dietary fiber in that great sweet tasting apple is just a bonus.

8. <u>Roasted Almonds</u> – Great taste, low sugar, high protein and high fiber makes this a great tasting and filling snack... there are many varieties available and if you want a great taste with a touch of sweetness, try the Emerald brand Cocoa Roast Almonds. For a mild salty taste, try the Sunkist brand Oven Roasted Almonds with Sea Salt… both very low sugar and very good for you!

9. <u>Tossed Salad with Original Fiber One</u> - Fresh lettuce, sliced tomatoes, carrot slices, grated cheese of any variety, but use the Original Fiber One cereal for your croutons to add lots of fiber and zero sugar. But, you have to be careful with the salad dressings… always carefully read the salad dressing label… and do not buy into the salad dressing low fat labeling… as you will find that many of the low fat dressings loaded with sugar. Most oil and vinegar or vinegarette varieties are very low sugar, but again, always check the label for grams of sugar. My personal favorite brand is "Newman's Own" Family Recipe Italian Dressing.

10. <u>Sliced Meats</u> - Ham, turkey and chicken are my favorites, or whatever meat appeals to you… there is no sugar here and high protein. Add a slice of Swiss or other cheese to the meat for a great filling high protein no-sugar snack.

11. <u>Eggs</u> – Enjoy Omelets, of almost any variety (but without the potatoes), Ham and Eggs, or Bacon and Eggs, for a great satisfying and filling meal, with very low sugar and high protein. Enjoy these with whole grain toast and peanut butter (but never with the little high sugar jam or jelly packets, and know you can ask for, and usually get, sugar free packets). Also recall there is no law that says you can only have these items for breakfast. Also, a quick, no sugar, high protein snack is to prepare microwave scrambled eggs by merely scrambling up 1 or 2 eggs in a cup, add 1 tablespoon water per egg, and cook until scrambled (usually 1 – 2 minutes). Go to "Google" and enter search: **microwave scrambled egg** for simple instructions.

12. <u>Shrimp Cocktail</u> – Enjoy this high protein, great filling sugar free item as an appetizer or a full meal, but be sure to use the sugar free cocktail sauce. The Walden Farms brand is a very good sugar free cocktail sauce. Further, when you have guests over for the big game, or whatever, put a batch of these out along with sliced meats, cheeses, and high fiber low sugar crackers. Your guests will be delighted as they enjoy your very healthy snacks.

In closing, you have to be diligent in your selection of snacks and drinks only with regard to the sugar content. Many retailers now offer a wide selection of sugar free "treats" with various dark chocolate and milk chocolate selections, along with many other varieties from which to choose. These, and many other satisfying sugar free items are locally available from multiple companies, including Hershey's, Russell Stover, Dove (Mars, Incorporated), and others. Further, go to "Google" and enter search: **sugar free food** and you will find a wide variety of quality sugar free products.

Further, based on your new understanding of the essential need to avoid refined sugar to lose weight and help lower your cholesterol, you need to become an avid label reader, to look for lowest sugar and highest dietary fiber. Remember "MISS" - <u>M</u>ake <u>I</u>t <u>S</u>hort & <u>S</u>imple and SOS – <u>S</u>top <u>O</u>nly <u>S</u>ugar.

APPENDIX B - SUGAR IN POPULAR SOFT DRINKS

Always remember what your body does with the refined sugar you drink or eat → STORE IT AS BODY FAT !

TEASPOONS OF SUGAR CONTENT IN:			
Product	12 oz:	20 oz:	Grams of Refined Sugar per 20 oz*
Water	0.0	0.0	0.0
Coca-Cola	9.3	15.4	77.0
Diet Coca-Cola	0.0	0.0	0.0
Coke Zero	0.0	0.0	0.0
Diet Rite (all varieties)	0.0	0.0	0.0
Pepsi	9.8	16.3	81.5
Diet Pepsi	0.0	0.0	0.0
Dr. Pepper	9.5	15.8	79.0
Diet Dr. Pepper	0.0	0.0	0.0
Barq's Root Beer	10.7	17.8	89.0
Diet Barq's Root Beer	0.0	0.0	0.0
Mountain Dew	11.0	18.3	91.5
Diet Mountain Dew	0.0	0.0	0.0
Sprite	9.0	14.9	74.5
Diet Sprite	0.0	0.0	0.0
Orange Slice	11.9	19.8	99.0
Minute Maid Soda	11.9	19.8	99.0
Hawaiian Fruit Punch	10.2	16.9	84.5
Squirt	9.5	15.8	79.0
Diet Squirt	0.0	0.0	0.0
Nestea	5.0	8.3	41.5
Diet Nestea	0.0	0.0	0.0
Gatorade	5.3	8.8	44.0

*ONE TEASPOON = 5 GRAMS OF REFINED SUGAR

Appendix C

IRRITABLE BOWEL SYNDROME (IBS)

What is Irritable Bowel Syndrome?

Irritable Bowel Syndrome, or IBS, is a very common disorder of the digestive tract. It affects the colon, or large intestine, usually over a long period of time. An estimated 30 million people in the USA, two thirds of whom are women, suffer from IBS. IBS is not a disease, and should not be confused with ulcerative colitis. Through the years, IBS has been called by many names such as "nervous" colon, mucous colitis, spastic colon, colitis, spastic bowel, and functional bowel disease. Most of these terms are inaccurate. The term "colitis" should never be used to define IBS.

What are the symptoms of IBS?

The term "syndrome" refers to a set of symptoms that occur together. The symptoms of IBS include abdominal pain, gas, bloating, a change in bowel habits, diarrhea, constipation, or constipation alternating with diarrhea. Rectal bleeding is never a symptom of IBS.

What causes IBS?

It is believed that most of the symptoms of IBS occur when the muscles in the colon do not work properly. The role of the colon, or large intestine, is to act as the waste disposal system of the body and to absorb water from the liquid stool that enters it from the small intestine. The stool then passes to the rectum where it is stored until a bowel movement occurs. The process is controlled by nerves and the muscles of the wall of the colon. In people with IBS, the muscles of the colon contract abnormally. An abnormal contraction, or spasm, may speed up the passage of stool, resulting in diarrhea. At other times, the spasm may delay the passage of stool, resulting in constipation. The exact cause of IBS is unknown. However, it may be associated with emotional stress or a low fiber diet.

How is IBS treated?

Once your doctor has determined that you have IBS and not a more serious disease, he or she will work closely with you to recommend effective treatment for your IBS. Adding fiber to your diet has clearly been shown to lessen or eliminate IBS symptoms. Dietary fiber is something you ingest (eat) that you cannot digest. The fiber passes through the stomach, through the small intestine and into the colon (large intestine). The fiber then absorbs water and liquid in the colon. If you have diarrhea, the fiber will absorb the extra water and fluid and will make for less frequent and more formed bowel movements. If you have constipation, the fiber will soften the stool and increase your number of bowel movements. Fiber also decreases the pressure in the colon. If needed, your doctor may also recommend anti-diarrhea medications that have been shown to be very effective in treating the severe diarrhea symptoms of IBS.

Can IBS lead to more serious problems?

IBS has not been shown to lead to any serious disease such as colitis or cancer. All patients with IBS should work closely with their physician to lessen their IBS symptoms. By establishing effective communication with your physician, Irritable Bowel Syndrome can be very effectively managed.

APPENDIX D

DIVERTICULOSIS AND DIVERTICULITIS

WHAT IS DIVERTICULOSIS?

Diverticulosis is a condition in which pouches (or small sacs) form on the wall of the large intestine or colon. The pouches are usually about ½ inch or less in size, and are found most often on the left side of the colon. Most people with diverticulosis do not have any symptoms at all and they may never know they have the condition. <u>With diverticulosis, you do NOT have to avoid seeds, nuts, popcorn, peanuts, berries, or any specific foods at all</u>. A high fiber diet is recommended.

WHAT IS DIVERTICULITIS?

The term "divertic<u>ulitis</u>" refers to an infected or inflamed pouch. The term "itis" on the end of a medical word means inflammation or infection. People with diverticulitis usually feel left-sided abdominal pain. People with diverticulitis <u>need</u> to be treated with antibiotics, usually as an out-patient, but more serious cases may need hospitalization and I.V. antibiotics.

HOW ARE THESE DISORDERS DIAGNOSED?

Most often diverticu<u>losis</u> causes no symptoms and is discovered by an x-ray or intestinal examination done for an unrelated reason. The doctor may see the diverticula (pouches) on an x-ray or during a colonoscopy procedure. Patients experiencing the symptoms of diverticu<u>litis</u> with left-sided abdominal pain, often with a fever, should see their physician as soon as possible to determine what is causing the symptoms.

HOW COMMON ARE THESE DISORDERS?

Diverticulosis is very common, especially in older adults. Studies show that about 10% of Americans over age 40 have diverticulosis, and greater than 50% over age 60. However, only about 20% of patients with diverticulosis ever have any problems such as diverticulitis.

ARE THESE DISORDERS SERIOUS?

For most people, diverticul<u>osis</u> is not a problem. Diverticul<u>itis</u> is a serious medical condition. An infected or inflamed pouch can lead to serious infection called an abscess, or a hole (perforation) in the bowel wall. People experiencing symptoms should always see their physician without delay for a proper diagnosis and treatment plan.

HOW ARE DIVERTICULOSIS AND DIVERTICULITIS TREATED?

If you have diverticulosis with no symptoms, treatment is not required, but it is a good idea to generally follow a high fiber diet. Fiber-rich foods such as whole grain cereals and breads, fruits and vegetables, and other high fiber foods reduce pressure in the colon and promote a healthy digestive tract with a normal bowel pattern. Laxatives and enemas should <u>not</u> be used regularly. Patients with diverticulitis should be promptly treated with antibiotics and possibly dietary restrictions. Severe cases may require hospitalization and possible surgery. Your physician can discuss diverticulosis and diverticulitis with you in greater detail.

APPENDIX E – COLORECTAL CANCER SCREENING GUIDELINES

Colorectal cancer is the second leading cause of cancer death in the United States and is one of the <u>most preventable</u> human cancers. Colorectal cancer is appropriately called the "silent killer" because most patients usually have no early symptoms. In fact, the most common <u>early</u> symptom of colon cancer is <u>nothing</u> at all. Therefore, do not believe that if you are having no symptoms and feeling well, that you should not have colorectal cancer screening. So the bad news is that colorectal cancer is common, but the good news is that this cancer is almost totally preventable with colorectal cancer screening. Colorectal cancer is curable if diagnosed and treated early. For screening, a colonoscopy is recommended for all persons over 50 years of age even if they have no symptoms. With a family history of colon cancer, colonoscopy should be done at age 40.

Almost all colorectal cancer develops from polyps, which are small benign but pre-cancerous growths on the inner lining of the colon. These polyps are common and generally are present in the colon or rectum with absolutely no symptoms. Therefore, the vast majority of people with these polyps are not aware they have polyps. Screening in the form of a colonoscopy is the standard of care. It is a safe, effective, painless method of visually examining the entire colon and rectum while the patient is sedated. Polyps are removed during the colonoscopy examination and any other potential abnormal findings can be checked at that time.

Guideline Summary: A colonoscopy should be done at 50 years of age even if a patient has no symptoms and at age 40 with a family history of colon cancer. Of course, if any symptoms at all - such as rectal bleeding, a change in bowel habits, unexplained symptoms such as weight loss, abdominal pain, or anemia - you should be checked right away. A colonoscopy should be performed every 5-10 years thereafter if no abnormalities are found. If polyps are found, or with a family history of colorectal cancer or polyps, more frequent examinations are recommended. Be certain to discuss this very important colorectal cancer screening with your personal health care provider.

(Sources: American Cancer Society, American Society of Colon and Rectal Surgeons)

APPENDIX F - WHEN SMOKERS QUIT

JUST 20 minutes after you've smoked that last cigarette, your body begins an ongoing series of beneficial changes:

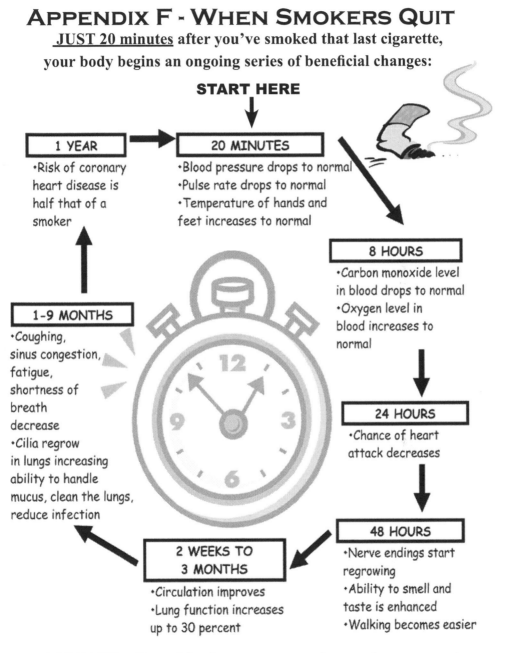

START HERE

20 MINUTES
•Blood pressure drops to normal
•Pulse rate drops to normal
•Temperature of hands and feet increases to normal

1 YEAR
•Risk of coronary heart disease is half that of a smoker

8 HOURS
•Carbon monoxide level in blood drops to normal
•Oxygen level in blood increases to normal

1-9 MONTHS
•Coughing, sinus congestion, fatigue, shortness of breath decrease
•Cilia regrow in lungs increasing ability to handle mucus, clean the lungs, reduce infection

24 HOURS
•Chance of heart attack decreases

48 HOURS
•Nerve endings start regrowing
•Ability to smell and taste is enhanced
•Walking becomes easier

2 WEEKS TO 3 MONTHS
•Circulation improves
•Lung function increases up to 30 percent

IMPORTANT - Post this sheet on your mirror where you get ready every morning, and read it every day without fail! It will program your subconscious mind, and we have had hundreds of patients quit with this simple yet effective technique.

SOS DIET GLOSSARY OF COMMON DIETARY MEDICAL TERMS

Body Mass Index (BMI) - BMI is calculated, or taken from a chart, based on a person's height and weight. This BMI number is then used to define underweight (less than 18.5), normal weight (18.5 to 24.9), overweight (25 to 29.9) or obese (30 or greater). Using BMI numbers for the USA, 2/3 of adults over age 20 and 1/3 of children age 2 to 19 are considered overweight or obese.

Cholesterol – Cholesterol is a complex biochemical substance considered to be a steroid and is essential to sustain human life. It is found in all human cell walls, and used in our body to manufacture our internal steroids, hormones, vitamin D, and bile. The vast majority of cholesterol in the human body is manufactured in the liver and only a small percentage of cholesterol comes from dietary intake of cholesterol.

Dietary Fiber – Dietary fiber is generally from plants and cannot be digested. It absorbs fluid, adds bulk to the stools, decreases pressure in the colon, and promotes healthy passage of waste material through the human digestive system. Because of the actions of dietary fiber, it is used to treat diarrhea, constipation, diverticulosis, Irritable Bowel Syndrome, lower cholesterol, and prevent colorectal cancer. A high fiber diet is generally considered to contain about 30 grams of dietary fiber per day.

Glycemic Index (GI) – The GI is a number based on the rise in blood sugar from ingesting 50 grams of pure glucose, and this is given the basis number of 100. Other foods are then ranked based on their specific effect on the blood glucose level. The glycemic index uses a scale of 0 to 100, with higher values given to foods that cause higher blood sugar levels and resulting higher insulin levels.

HDL Cholesterol – HDL stands for high-density lipoprotein, and is considered to be your "good" cholesterol. It is believed that HDL can remove built-up plaque from arteries. Therefore a high level of this HDL cholesterol helps to protect against cardiovascular disease. It is reported as the separate HDL value on cholesterol laboratory work.

LDL Cholesterol – LDL stands for low-density lipoprotein, and is considered to be your "bad" cholesterol. It is believed the elevated levels of LDL promote the formation of arterial plaque, and is therefore associated with atherosclerosis, leading to potential heart attacks, stroke, and peripheral vascular disease. It is also reported as a separate value on laboratory work to check for blood cholesterol levels.

Net Carbs – This is a simple formula to calculate the "net" effect of carbohydrate grams in a specific food on your insulin production. The nets carbs value is equal to the total carbohydrate (TC) grams minus dietary fiber (DF) grams minus one half the sugar alcohol (SA) grams, or as follows: (TC – DF - ½ SA = Net Carbs).

Omega-3 Fatty Acid – These are unsaturated fats and therefore are considered to be the healthy dietary fats. There is scientific evidence that regular intake will reduce the risk of heart attack, stroke, and build-up of plaque in the arteries. They also have been shown to reduce elevated blood triglyceride levels and may help reduce blood pressure. However, if taken to excess, there may be harmful side effects, such as prolonged bleeding. Specific dietary recommendations should be discussed with your health care provider.

Probiotics – The probiotics are dietary supplements containing live bacterial and yeast microorganisms to add these organisms to the human digestive tract and are used to treat a deficiency of these organisms. This is not a new concept as they were originally described in the early 1900's.

Saturated Fats – Saturated fat is dietary fat that is made up of triglycerides containing only saturated fatty acids. The term saturated means that these fatty acid chains are fully saturated with hydrogen atoms. The true extent to which saturated fats may be healthy or unhealthy is continually being questioned and research is ongoing. Be aware that there are conflicting reports in the literature as to the true impact of saturated fats on one's health.

Sugar Alcohols – Sugar alcohols are naturally occurring substances that are found in plants, sugar and starches. They taste sweet, but have the advantage that they are not readily absorbed by the body. Therefore, unlike refined sugar, they are not stored as fat and have less impact on blood sugar levels and only minimal impact on blood cholesterol. Dental research has also shown that sugar alcohols do not promote tooth decay. Be aware that if sugar alcohols are consumed in large quantities, they may have a laxative effect and promote diarrhea. This laxative effect is uncommon and clearly depends on the quantity consumed.

Trans Fats – These are the unhealthy fats in your diet. Trans fats are partially hydrogenated oils and this process was developed to convert a liquid fat into a solid or semi-solid fat. They have been in our diet since the early 1900's. It is now well established that eating trans fats increases one's risk of heart disease because trans fats raise levels of "bad" LDL cholesterol and lowering levels of "good" HDL cholesterol. Dietary trans fats should be avoided and fortunately, they are becoming more and more difficult to find.

Triglycerides – Triglycerides are so named because they consist of three fatty acids attached to a molecule of glycerol (a chemical alcohol). The type of attached fatty acids will vary and may be saturated, monounsaturated, or polyunsaturated fatty acids. They play an important role in human metabolism as energy sources and transporters of dietary fat. The blood carries the triglycerides throughout your body to give you energy or to be stored as body fat. The exact role of elevated triglyceride levels as a specific cause of disease is not clear but may be associated with heart disease and research is ongoing. Elevated triglyceride levels often result from excess alcohol use and may also be associated with pancreatitis.

Unsaturated Fats – These are considered to be the healthy fats in your diet. The three main types are polyunsaturated fats, monounsaturated fats, and omega-3 fatty acids. Unsaturated fats are proven to be "heart-healthy" because they tend to decrease total cholesterol, increase HDL cholesterol, and lower LDL cholesterol.

INDEX

NEED MORE COPIES OF
SOS DIET - STOP ONLY SUGAR?

EASY WAYS TO ORDER

1. ORDER ON-LINE AT – www.sosdietbook.com

2. MAIL check and a copy of this order form to:

Bean Books, LLC, 416 W. Ave. B, Newberry, MI 49868

Name_____

Title_____

Organization _____

Shipping address _____

City_____ State_____ Zip_____

Phone _____ Fax_____

PRICE INCLUDES FREE SHIPPING – ORDER NOW

SOS Diet Book _____ Copies X $19.95 = $ _____

For Michigan shipping address,
add 6% Sales Tax ($1.20 per book) $ _____

Total (U. S. Dollars) $ _____

– PAYMENT –

☐ **Check enclosed** (Make Payable to Bean Books)

Quantity discounts available.

– QUESTIONS –
Contact James A. Surrell M.D.
via e-mail: sosdietdoc@gmail.com

ABOUT THE AUTHOR

James A. Surrell M. D. is a board-certified colorectal surgeon and holds fellowship status in the American Society of Colon and Rectal Surgeons and the American College of Surgeons. He devoted 14 years to formal education with 4 years of pre-med at Northern Michigan University, 4 years of medical school at Michigan State University, 5 years of general surgery residency and one year of colorectal surgery fellowship... (Whew)! He has been a practicing colorectal surgeon for the past 20 plus years. Dr. Surrell has authored many articles in various journals on topics related to his specialty of colorectal surgery and digestive health.

He has a special interest in nutrition and weight loss programs. As Director of the Digestive Health Institute, his practice is focused on digestive health, including nutrition, dietary weight management and colorectal cancer screening and prevention. He is known in his large practice for his ability to communicate effectively with his patients, and he goes to great lengths not to speak "doctor talk" to his patients.

"Doc" or Jim (as he prefers to be called) is also a much sought-after speaker. He speaks frequently to local, regional, and national public and professional groups. He blends a significant amount of humor into his many talks and is generally available to speak to nearly any group with an interest in learning more about various topics, including: diet and weight loss, nutrition, cancer prevention, and other healthy lifestyle topics. He also appears frequently on his local "Ask the Doctors" program on Public TV. Here is your author's favorite quote:

"There isn't much humor in medicine,
but there's a lot of medicine in humor."

Dr. Jim feels very strongly that for any weight loss program to be successful, it must be short, simple and easy to understand. Thus was born the SOS Diet – Stop Only Sugar and the "MISS" (Make It Short & Simple) concept. This short and simple SOS Diet has worked so very well for him and for so many of his patients, friends and colleagues for years. He is now most appreciative of this opportunity to present it to you in the form of this short and simple SOS Diet book.

Good luck and SOS - Stop Only Sugar!

Made in the USA
Lexington, KY
29 July 2010